The
Home
Herbal

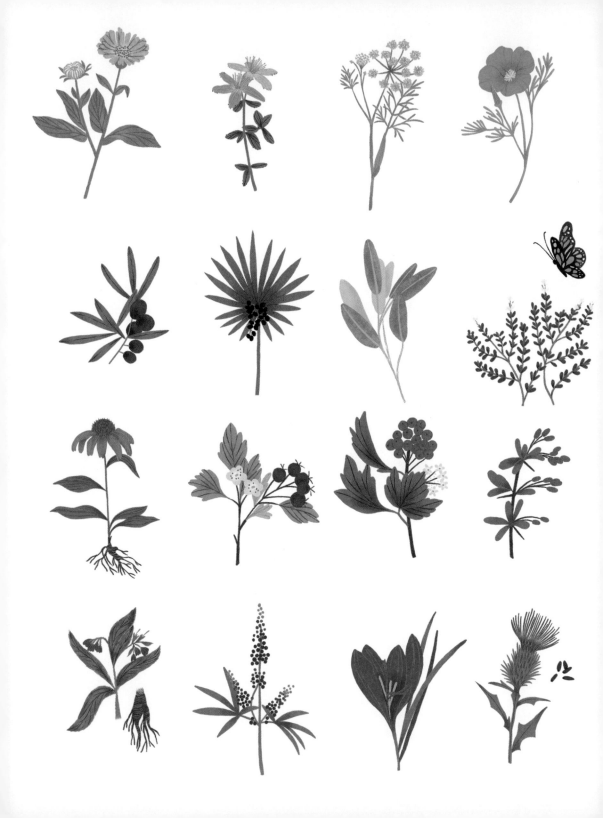

The
Home
Herbal

Restorative herbal
recipes for the mind,
body, and soul

Andrew Chevallier FNIMH, MCPP

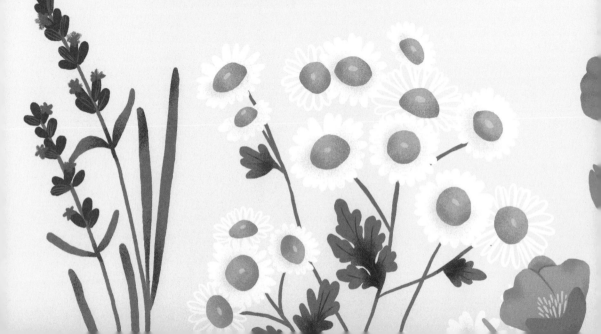

Introduction

Herbal medicine has been used since the earliest times to heal and cure. The natural world provides tens of thousands of plant remedies that work to relieve illness and restore health and well-being. The tradition of herbal knowledge being passed down from one generation to another is a rarity now. Herbal knowledge comes via the written word, whether from a book or the internet, and each year research brings fresh insights into plant medicines, expanding our understanding and their potential range of use. The problem now is that there is often no one at hand able to give the advice and support needed to use herbal medicines successfully and with confidence.

As a self-care book, *The Home Herbal* seeks to fill this gap and to provide the advice and support to enable readers to treat day-to-day health problems with herbal medicine safely and effectively. As a "home" herbal, it is a practical book to use when minor accidents or family illness require it, and it provides clear instructions on how to heal or relieve more than 100 common ailments: everyday problems such as cuts, grazes, headaches, and sore throats; emotional health issues such as anxiety, irritability, and stress; as well as more serious or long-term ailments such as arthritis, chronic cystitis, high blood pressure, and shingles.

Caring for yourself, or for someone else, is not easy; it takes time, commitment, and perseverance. *The Home Herbal* helps you to make sense of ill health and to question what might lie behind it. Identifying symptoms and placing them in context, and understanding what is needed for healing and recovery to take place, gives you a better chance of finding effective natural treatments to aid recovery and speed the return of good health and well-being. Simple suggestions are also made throughout the book to support emotional health and balance – a prerequisite for robust physical health – as well as pointers to relieve the anxiety and distress that often accompanies ill health.

Despite all this, *The Home Herbal* is a book and not more – it cannot replace the advice and treatment of an experienced healthcare provider. If you or someone you are caring for is seriously unwell or you feel out of your depth in treating yourself or someone else, please do seek professional advice. See Being Unwell (pp. 16–23).

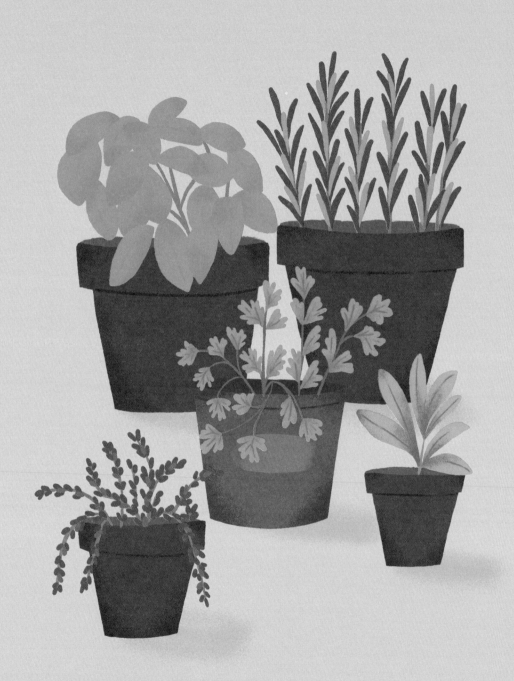

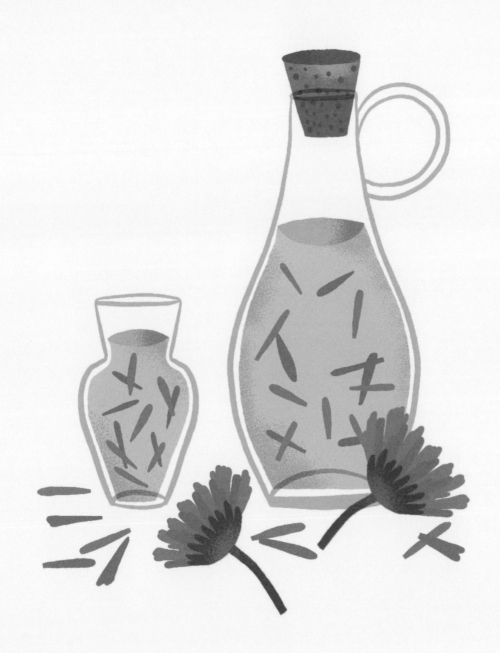

LEARNING TO USE HERBAL MEDICINE

You can use *The Home Herbal* as printed herbals have always been used – that is, pick it up when you need it and leaf through it to find helpful remedies to alleviate health complaints of all kinds. The book is a reference guide that links symptoms, ailments, and ill health to specific herbal remedies, giving detailed advice on herbal combinations, how best to use them, dosages, and cautions. The recommended treatments in Chapter 4: Common Ailments – for nausea, for example – can be cross-referenced with Chapter 5: Herb Profiles, allowing you to review the wider options and so gain a greater depth of understanding in using herbal remedies.

You simply look up a condition in Chapter 4: Common Ailments and take note of the suggested remedies – in the case of nausea, the main herbs listed are chamomile, lavender, peppermint, and ginger. Each herb has a profile in Chapter 5, with more information on the conditions it treats, the best ways to take it, and at what dosage. You will notice that not all of the herbs listed in the remedies in Chapter 4 feature in Chapter 5, in which case they are set in italic. On pp. 248–249, an index of herbs lists all of the herbs used in the book alphabetically by their common names, together with their scientific names. This will ensure that you source the correct herbs when buying them.

Reading the book straight through from cover to cover will give you a broad understanding of herbal medicine and self-care, detailed knowledge of recommended self-treatment choices and of key herbal medicines, along with guidance about using and making herbal remedies safely and effectively. You will learn about herbal medicine and develop confidence in using herbs on a regular basis.

If you prefer to read different sections as they become relevant or of interest to you, your herbal knowledge will grow like a kind of mosaic. As far as possible, the experience of being ill has been given equal weight to the description of what ill health looks like and signifies in terms of symptoms. Both, when combined, give you the best chance of arriving at effective self-treatment.

Chapter 6: Using Herbal Medicines Wisely covers how to prepare and make your own herbal medicines and includes instructions for using them safely and effectively. You will also find advice on what to include in your own home herbal medicine chest, and a list of suggestions for the best medicinal plants to grow at home – in a garden, on a balcony, or on a windowsill – so that you can grow, make, and then use your own herbal remedies.

SAFETY AND EFFECTIVENESS

An ever-expanding body of research over the last 40 years or so has shown that medicinal plants – particularly those with longstanding traditional use – have immense therapeutic value. Herbs such as ginkgo, Korean ginseng, and St John's wort have become commonly used remedies and their value as medicines has been scientifically validated. While the herbs recommended in *The Home Herbal* have all been the subject of research, their effectiveness as medicines is not yet fully established scientifically. Nevertheless, herbs such as nettle and olive leaf have been used successfully as traditional medicines over thousands of years and have an extremely high safety profile. As our collective knowledge of a plant's activity within the body grows, so a clearer picture emerges of how it may act as a medicine and how it can be best used therapeutically.

In herbal medicine, the effectiveness of a remedy depends on the quality of the ingredients, on the type of preparation – such as infusion, tincture, or powder – and on the dosage. All these are of singular importance – if poor-quality material is used, if the herbs are processed in an inappropriate way, or taken at the wrong dosage, the effectiveness, and possibly the safety, of the remedy may be compromised. In short, quality is essential to herbal medicine.

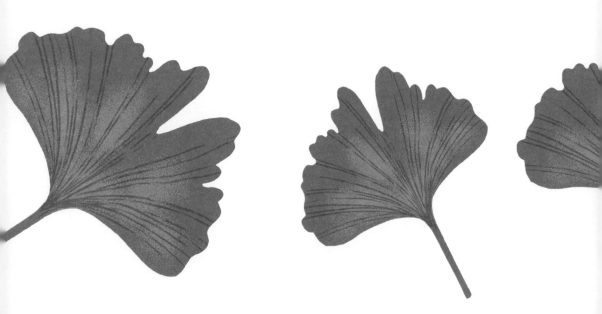

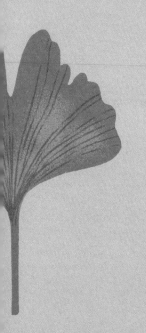

All the advice and information you will need to navigate your way through these sometimes complex quality issues can be found in Chapter 6: Using Herbal Medicines Wisely. All suggested treatments throughout the book include recommended dosages. Additionally, Chapter 5: Herb Profiles lists the best preparations and recommended dosage for each herb. Although such quality concerns do not generally apply to manufactured herbal remedies, which should have undergone rigorous quality control, not all manufactured products are exactly what they claim to be. Adulteration is not uncommon, especially where more costly herbs are concerned. Pointers towards sourcing good-quality products are also given in Chapter 6.

All the herbs recommended in this book are known to be safe when used correctly; many of them, such as ginger and rosemary, are well-known spices and dietary ingredients. When used appropriately, they carry a minimal risk of side-effects. In rare circumstances, side-effects can occur – typically a mild headache, digestive upset, or diarrhoea. Such symptoms almost invariably clear on stopping treatment.

Relief of symptoms can be slower with plant remedies, although there are grounds for thinking that recovery when taking herbal remedies tends to be more enduring. Detailed advice on cautions and safe use is given for each herb in Chapter 5 and throughout Chapter 6.

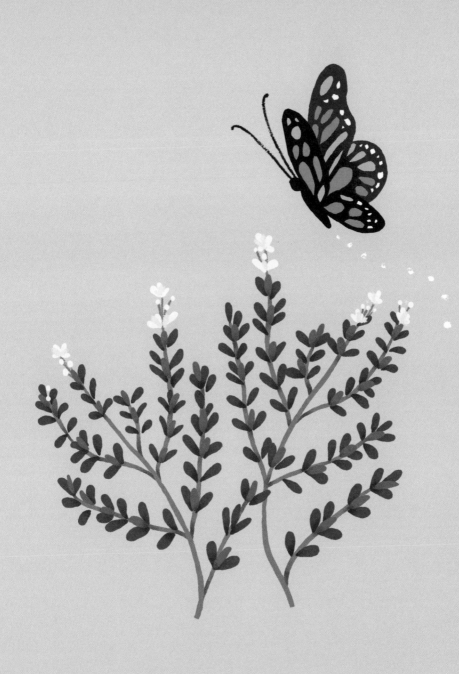

ENVIRONMENTAL IMPACT

Medicinal plants, like all native plants, are an intrinsic part of the natural world. Until relatively recently, most medicinal plants were gathered locally from wild meadows, forests, and mountains across the planet. When a plant is collected on a small scale for use personally and within communities, the native plant population is protected, as the community has a direct interest in ensuring its continued survival. However, when medicinal plants are collected commercially from the wild in an uncontrolled way, specific medicinal plants can be threatened to the point of extinction. Plants such as echinacea, once common across the prairies, are now rare in the wild due to commercial overexploitation, though paradoxically, echinacea species are now common garden plants. This is a complex issue with a long history. For example, while the first recorded case of extinction of a medicinal plant – silphion, a carrot family member – occurred in the 1st century CE, herbs and spices such as cinnamon and cloves have been traded for about 3,000 years.

Most medicinal plants are now cultivated commercially rather than gathered from the wild. When you are purchasing dried herbs and manufactured remedies, buy ones that have been cultivated organically or in a certified responsible manner. Medicinal plants harvested from the wild in an environmentally sustainable manner should be certified as such. Many medicinal plants, including black cohosh and rhodiola, are still threatened by overexploitation.

The most sustainable way to use herbs, of course, is to grow them organically yourself in a garden, backyard, or balcony and harvest them for use, either fresh or dried. Not only does this minimize the herbs' environmental footprint but it supports insect life and soil quality. Some herbs such as melissa and thyme are especially attractive to bees and butterflies.

HEALING AND PLANT LIFE

Our lives are interwoven with the plant world in an almost infinite number of ways. In common with all animal life, we depend for our sustenance directly or indirectly on the leaves, roots, seeds, and fruits that the natural world provides. Plants are also a main source of medicine, of materials for construction, of cloth, clothes, and so on. These key connections with the plant world are all practical, they all serve a purpose. *The Home Herbal* is a further example of this interrelationship.

But there is a way of relating to the plant world that is not purposive, that involves the heart as much as the head. The beauty of a sunflower, the scent of honeysuckle on a summer morning, the stark, coolness of a forest in winter – these connections, these delights, enrich our lives and open us up to the healing power of nature.

Hospital patients recover more quickly if they can see trees and greenery from their window. Sitting surrounded by plants in a garden or among trees in woodland also calms the mind and brings a sense of quiet joy. Opening up to this aspect of the plant world is not a part of herbal medicine in itself, but when you next sit drinking a herbal infusion or swallow a herbal capsule or tablet, remember where it came from.

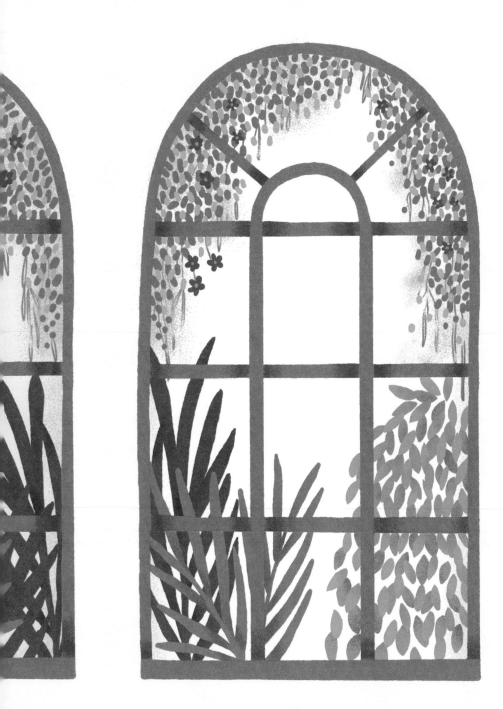
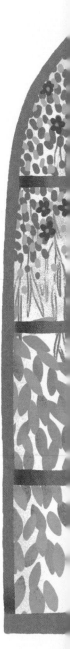

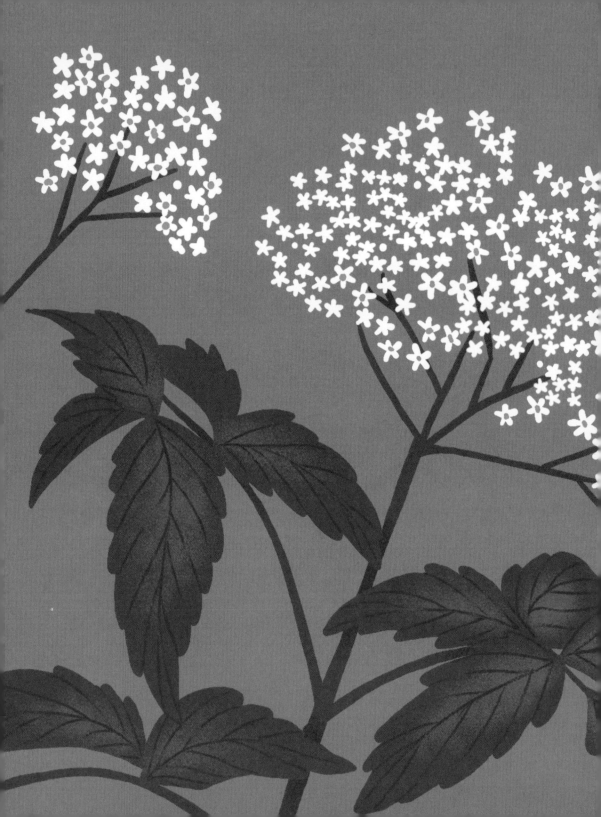

Being Unwell

In this chapter, you will find information about key signs and symptoms that are associated with serious illness. Whenever you are unwell, it makes good sense to ask yourself whether your symptoms are sufficiently worrying that you need to be assessed by a healthcare practitioner or whether you can safely treat yourself.

1

Being Unwell

Ill health can be hard to make sense of – it ranges all the way from the minor discomfort of a cold sore or mouth ulcer to life-threatening disease. Symptoms can be difficult to interpret and working out what to do when unwell can be a challenge.

Feeling unwell means coping with both unwanted, unpleasant symptoms and with the anxiety that undiagnosed ill health can cause. As much as a book can, *The Home Herbal* aims to help you take a calm, informed look at your symptoms when ill, and to work out how best to care for and treat yourself with herbal medicines, banishing anxiety and making a speedy recovery. As a self-help book, it is important to emphasize, however, that there are limits to how far you can successfully treat yourself. Somewhere within the terrain of ill health is a none-too-well defined boundary line that divides those health problems suitable for home treatment and self-care from more serious ill health that requires the input of a healthcare professional, whether as a matter of common sense or as an emergency.

This chapter looks at signs and symptoms that are potentially worrisome and lists "red flag" signs that warn if you or someone in your care has crossed this boundary line and may be seriously unwell. If you find you have symptoms that match a "red flag" sign (see pp. 22–23) or if you feel seriously unwell, you might be able to treat this problem yourself, but it is far better and more reassuring to have someone experienced in dealing with health issues assess you and give you the advice and treatment that you need.

In the far more likely situation that your symptoms are mild or moderate and come nowhere near the threshold of serious illness, you can, if you want, skip to Chapter 2: Understanding Health and Illness, which explores key factors that underpin health and gives pointers to herbal remedies and treatment.

MAJOR SIGNS AND SYMPTOMS

The common signs and symptoms briefly considered here are ones that most people have experienced at one time or another. Their significance lies in the fact that, if unchecked or left uncontrolled, they can lead to serious or life-threatening illness, so do take notice if they occur.

FEVER

By and large, fever is a positive sign. It occurs when the body's thermostat sets a higher temperature than normal, usually in response to a viral or bacterial infection. Fever enables the body's metabolism to work faster, speeding up all aspects of immune function, stimulating sweating, and shortening the time taken to recovery. At temperatures up to 39°C (102°F), bedrest, lots of liquids, a watchful eye, and gentle supportive remedies are what are needed. If the temperature rises above 40°C (104°F), or if a fever lasts for more than three days, you should contact your healthcare practitioner. To bring down a fever, wrap wet towels on the body or take a cooling bath. A vinegar compress helps to stimulate sweating.

+ See Colds and Flu (p. 103)

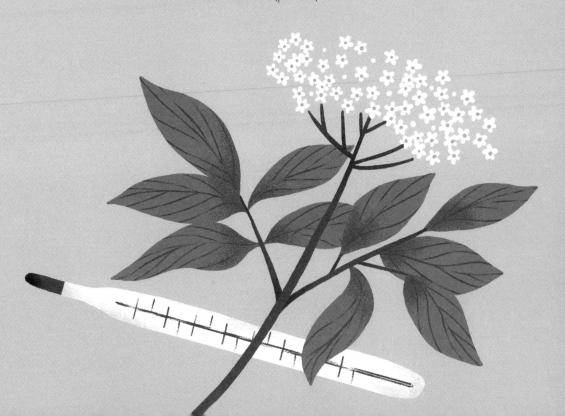

PAIN	A powerful call to attend to the painful site, pain plays a protective role. Sudden severe pain or ongoing chronic pain – for example, in the chest – demands urgent medical investigation. Pain can be felt far from the site producing the pain (described as referred pain), making it hard to interpret. In mild or moderate pain, having some idea of the type of pain involved and the factors causing it can help in identifying effective pain relief and treatment. + See Understanding Pain (p. 40)
BREATHING PROBLEMS	Problems with breathing vary from mild breathlessness to severe breathing difficulty. Minor breathing problems due to excess catarrh, acute anxiety, or a viral infection can generally be treated effectively with herbal medicines, however noticeable difficulty in breathing, for example in asthma or certain cases of Covid-19, requires immediate treatment. If you, or someone in your care, is struggling to breathe or has low blood oxygen levels (<94 per cent) seek immediate medical treatment. You can measure blood oxygen levels using a pulse oximeter on the fingertip – though note that physical signs of illness are more important than measurements. + See Painful Dry Coughs (p. 106); Asthma (p. 109)
VOMITING	This bodily response brings up the stomach contents and empties the stomach. When caused by infection or toxicity, the unpleasant experience of vomiting is usually followed by a sense of relief. Many other conditions, including migraine and travel sickness, cause vomiting, though here vomiting may be repeated unproductively with no sense of relief. If repeated nausea and vomiting occur without an identifiable cause, seek advice from your healthcare practitioner. + See Nausea and Vomiting (p. 113)
DIARRHOEA	A common problem, diarrhoea often indicates an imbalance in the gut flora (the microorganisms living in the digestive tract). Frequent, loose, or watery stools represent an attempt by the gut to clear irritants and toxins. Severe acute diarrhoea is dangerous because it leads to major fluid loss and dehydration, particularly in children. It needs emergency medical treatment. More manageable diarrhoea needs an increased fluid intake (2 litres/4 pints water a day) to compensate for fluid loss. Many factors, including emotional state and food sensitivity, can lie behind a pattern of

chronic diarrhoea, which is often given the catch-all diagnosis of irritable bowel syndrome (IBS).

+ See Diarrhoea, Looseness, and Urgency (p. 118)

HEART AND PULSE RATE	Changes in heart and pulse rate occur all the time in response to exercise, activity, and stress, to ensure that adequate blood flow reaches the tissues. At rest, the pulse rate (best taken at the wrist, known as your radial pulse) is typically 60–80 beats per minute depending on level of fitness, with 72 beats as an average. Athletes often have much lower rates. Resting pulse rates continuously above 100 or below 40 beats per minute need investigation. If you have palpitations and your heart rate becomes irregular or very fast, or you cannot feel a normal pulse and you feel breathless, contact your healthcare practitioner urgently.
BLEEDING AND BLOOD LOSS	External bleeding from a wound should stop within 10 minutes, once pressure has been applied consistently onto the site of the wound. If significant bleeding continues beyond this time, or if there has been significant blood loss, seek urgent medical advice. Key concerns relate to poor blood clotting – particularly in those taking anti-coagulant therapy, which prolongs the time taken for a clot to form – and to damage to a major blood vessel, which will require surgery to stop the bleed. Regular heavy menstrual bleeding may lead to anaemia, but an uncontrolled menstrual bleed needs urgent treatment. Internal bleeding may go unnoticed – bleeding within the gastrointestinal tract can produce an unusually dark stool (melaena).

+ See Cuts, Grazes, and Minor Wounds (p. 71) and Heavy Menstrual Bleeding (p. 141)

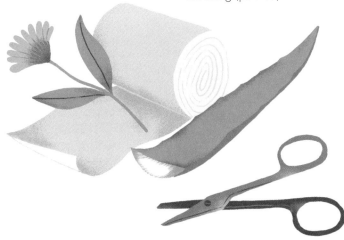

"RED FLAG" SIGNS

If one or more of these signs are present, make urgent contact with your healthcare practitioner or hospital department.

+ Fever above 39°C (102°F)
+ Severe pain of any kind, including back pain
+ Heavy nosebleed lasting more than one hour
+ Persistent one-sided headache, or headache that fails to improve within 48 hours
+ Severe depression
+ Loss of sensation or loss of movement
+ Difficulty in breathing or chest pain
+ Cough or hoarseness that lasts for more than three weeks
+ Palpitations lasting several minutes
+ Fainting or dizziness with weakness, numbness or tingling in any part of the body
+ Double vision/visual disturbance
+ Difficulty in swallowing
+ Infections that show no sign of improvement or deteriorate after taking herbal remedies
+ Vomiting blood
+ Blood in the stool
+ Pain in the kidneys
+ Blood in the urine
+ Significant or sudden change in menstruation, such as prolonged heavy or irregular bleeding
+ Postmenopausal bleeding more than one year after the last period
+ Sudden allergic reaction, including after taking a herbal remedy
+ Significant or sudden joint swelling or leg swelling
+ Lump in breast
+ Lump in testicle
+ Broken bones or any injury that may need an X-ray
+ Serious wounds, grazes, bruising, burns, bites, and stings

+ A mole that has changed shape, size, or colour, or itches or bleeds
+ A sore or boil that does not heal, or unexplained swellings beneath the skin
+ Shingles or suspected shingles

Children

Children can become ill very quickly but frequently recover as speedily as they get ill. If your child has any of the following signs or symptoms, make urgent contact with your healthcare practitioner or hospital department.

+ Severe vomiting or diarrhoea
+ Temperature over 39°C (102°F)
+ Fever with convulsions
+ Breathing difficulties
+ Unusual drowsiness
+ High-pitched crying

During pregnancy

Striking a healthy balance between ignoring symptoms that develop during pregnancy and being over-concerned about them can be difficult. Make urgent contact with your healthcare practitioner or hospital department should any of the following occur.

+ Prolonged nausea causing an inability to eat properly
+ Frequent vomiting leading to dehydration
+ Frequent urination lasting for more than three days (or with pain for two days)
+ Breast pain with swollen glands under the arms or fever
+ Fluid retention that has not reduced after three days

Understanding Health & Illness

This chapter looks at how the body works during times of well-being and illness, and in particular those factors that support good health and recovery from illness. It then gives practical advice about making sense of symptoms and pointers for treatment.

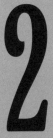

Maintaining Good Health

This section of the book takes a brief look at key physiological processes involved in maintaining health and defending the integrity of the body, and aims to provide an outline sketch of factors that commonly lie behind ill health. A better understanding of how our bodies work – in health and in illness – improves the chances of finding appropriate treatment and remedies. A list of key herbs relevant to each section is included and you can read about each in more detail in Chapter 5: Herb Profiles.

TISSUE HEALING AND REPAIR

The healing process is divided into four stages and effective healing depends on the completion of each stage in the following order: vasoconstriction, inflammation, proliferation, and remodelling (see opposite for a summary of each stage).

Many herbs help in each of these four stages of the healing process, controlling inflammation, reducing the risk of infection, and promoting effective healing. Some may also help to repair scar tissue. Working with your body and not placing excess demands on it will shorten the time taken to fully heal.

+ **Key herbs:** Aloe vera, arnica, marigold, chamomile, gotu kola, witch hazel, plantain, comfrey

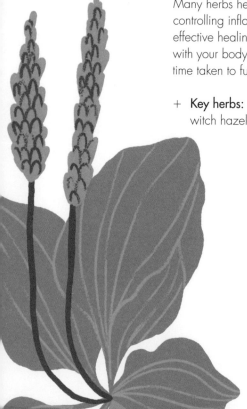

VASOCONSTRICTION

Blood vessels constrict to limit and stop bleeding, initiate clotting, and reduce the chances of infection occurring.

INFLAMMATION

Produces heat, swelling, and pain; the area is flooded with immune cells, such as macrophages, that mop up debris and counter infection.

REMODELLING

Scar tissue is formed, which in effective healing, gradually achieves the tensile and elastic quality of healthy skin.

PROLIFERATION

Granulation tissue rich in new blood cells is laid down and new skin tissue starts to form.

INFLAMMATION

Inflammation is a process that involves a powerful immune cell response to any damage, toxin, or infection that threatens the body's integrity. Effective inflammation neutralizes the threat, lays down the ground for the formation of new tissue, and ushers in the stages of healing that lead to full recovery.

Unfortunately, inflammation does not always lead to successful healing. If infection or toxicity is not effectively dealt with during the acute inflammatory stage, and continues to trigger an immune response, the healing process can become stuck in a state of chronic inflammation. In this ongoing situation, uncontrolled immune activity may last for several months or years and cause major tissue injury. Chronic inflammation is an underlying factor in many serious illnesses, including rheumatoid arthritis, fibromyalgia, psoriasis, and some cancers. It is also a key factor in ageing.

ACUTE INFLAMMATION	In acute inflammation, such as with a small wound, short-term treatment is needed to:
	+ clean the affected area and prevent infection; support and manage the inflammatory response; and stimulate the cell proliferation and remodelling that lead to tissue repair
	+ **Key herbs:** Aloe vera, arnica, marigold, *myrrh*, plantain, *tea tree*, comfrey
CHRONIC INFLAMMATION	In chronic inflammation, where the healing process has stalled and is stuck at the inflammatory stage, a different approach is needed to:
	+ manage and reduce inflammatory activity – locally and within the body as a whole; support effective immune function and treat underlying infection (if present); and stimulate all aspects of the healing process
	+ **Key herbs:** Aloe vera, chamomile, turmeric, liquorice, *willow bark*, ashwagandha, ginger

INFECTION AND IMMUNE FUNCTION

Our immune system is extraordinarily complex and involves the balanced interplay of many different types of white blood cells, signalling systems, and checks and balances. Its main role is to:

+ counter pathogens and remove them from the body

+ recognize and detoxify environmental toxins

+ cleanse damaged and cancerous cells

The inbuilt or innate part of the immune system, which implements the inflammatory processes looked at earlier, acts as a general defence against infection, attacking and mopping up infectious agents and toxins. The adaptive immune system, in contrast, produces antibodies that target and neutralize specific bacteria and viruses, even if they change over time.

Herbal medicines, such as echinacea and garlic, are known to enhance function in both arms of the immune system and to have anti-inflammatory activity. Tellingly, 75 per cent of the body's immune system is located in and around the walls of the gastrointestinal tract, the area within the body where infection is most likely to occur. Eating a healthy diet, including fermented foods and taking appropriate herbs, spices, and probiotics to support efficient digestion, absorption, and elimination is fundamental in maintaining a healthy immune system. Supporting healthy digestion and balanced immune function is essential in preventing and controlling chronic inflammation and auto-immune disease – both consequences of immune dysregulation.

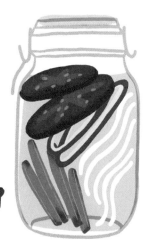

+ **Key herbs:** Garlic, barberry, *clove*, turmeric, echinacea, olive leaf, elderberry and flower, thyme, ginger

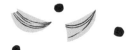

ALLERGY

Allergic reactions to irritants, such as pollen and cat hair, affect up to 20 per cent of the population, with the sneezing, runny nose, and sore eyes of hay fever or allergic rhinitis being the most common symptoms. Allergic reactions vary from discomfort and irritation to life-threatening anaphylactic shock, and while most allergies are relatively mild and manageable, more severe allergic reactions, such as peanut allergy and multiple wasp stings, require immediate medical intervention.

Allergies are caused by an over-sensitivity within the immune system that leads to histamine release in affected tissue, such as the skin or mucous membranes of the nose and eyes. Histamine is a powerful natural compound (it is present in nettle stings) that causes inflammation, swelling, pain, and the familiar red, sore, and swollen appearance of an allergic reaction. Common allergens include foods such as strawberries, milk, food additives such as tartrazine (E102), and sulphites, as well as insect stings, airborne particles, and handling certain plants – for example, ragwort.

The simplest treatment is to identify the allergen and minimize exposure to it – not always easy. Natural approaches can help, and the threshold that triggers an allergic response and the frequency and severity of symptoms can be improved.

+ **Key herbs:** Chamomile, liquorice, passion flower, elderflower, milk thistle, nettle leaf, valerian

TRY THIS

+ Keep well hydrated. Allergic reactions are stronger and more likely to occur when dehydrated.

+ Support liver health. Avoid deep-fried foods, junk food, dairy produce, sugar; eat more fruit and veg. Take milk thistle seeds or liquorice tincture.

+ Stress, worry, and anxiety increase histamine release, which in turn influences the frequency and strength of allergic reactions. Relaxation, mindfulness, and breathing exercises will help, as will calming herbs such as chamomile, passion flower, and valerian.

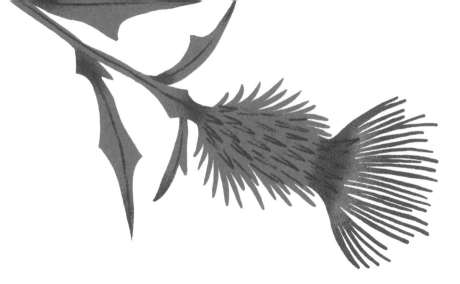

TOXICITY AND DETOXIFICATION

Good health depends as much on effective detoxification as it does on sound nutrition, and the clearance of waste products and toxins from the body by the liver and kidneys is essential to life. Water-soluble compounds are removed by the kidneys in the urine, other compounds are metabolized by the liver, pass through the bile ducts, and are removed in the faeces. Additionally, the body removes waste products in sweat, in mucus secretions, such as saliva, and via the lungs in breathing out.

Given these basic facts, it is apparent that any situation where toxicity is involved, whether it is eczema, gout, or environmental pollution, will get worse where dehydration (see Hydration, p. 32), a concentrated urine, poor bile flow, or chronic constipation (see Constipation, p. 117) are present. The starting point for treating toxicity of any kind is to stimulate kidney clearance and urine flow and establish regular bowel movements. Even upping fluid intake and eating more vegetables (especially fibrous roots) can make a significant difference.

The next stage involves enhancing liver metabolism and supporting the body in neutralizing inflammatory damage produced in response to toxins. In more severe cases, professional treatment is advisable but self-help treatment will often be effective, especially if pursued long-term.

+ **Key herbs:** Marigold, turmeric, artichoke, echinacea, olive leaf, milk thistle, dandelion, rosemary

HYDRATION

Human beings are not camels, we have no reserve tank to call on if we start to become dehydrated. We rarely think about it, but our bodies are made up of about 60 per cent water. Young babies are around 75 per cent water, while older adults are closer to 50 per cent water. These figures show quite starkly why good hydration is essential for good health – insufficient fluid within the body means poor delivery of nutrients to cells and sluggish removal of waste products.

Many health problems can be eased or cured simply by keeping well hydrated. As we age, it becomes harder for our bodies to retain water, so older adults are more prone to dehydration. Here is just a short list of symptoms that can result just from dehydration:

+ headache, confusion
+ tiredness and fatigue
+ dizziness, weakness, light-headedness
+ dry mouth and/or a dry cough
+ high heart rate but low blood pressure
+ loss of appetite
+ flushed skin, swollen feet, muscle cramps

People who start hydrating well after a prolonged period of under-hydration can find that their health is transformed simply with an increased fluid intake. Drinking roughly 2 litres (4 pints) of fluid a day, with at least half of this being water, is a "no-brainer". Many drinks, for example tea and coffee, are diuretic, so although body fluid levels are being topped up, the kidneys are also being stimulated to remove fluid. Water is the most effective drink in maintaining balanced fluid levels.

ADAPTIVE CAPACITY

Our bodies like internal stability and continuity more than anything else. These conditions enable the body to adapt and self-correct and maintain the body's inner environment in a steady state, no matter what demands are being placed on it in the outer world. Consistent body temperature, blood and fluid volume, acid/alkali balance, and hormonal function are some of the many factors that sustain this balanced internal functioning, known as homeostasis. In good health, the body has a remarkable capacity to deal with extreme demands or stresses – whether challenged by the outer world, for example extremes of heat or cold, or by fungal infection or heavy metal toxicity in the inner environment. Our bodies can adapt rapidly to minor or gradual change, but major change becomes stressful if it pushes the body close to or beyond its adaptive limits.

Anything that saps, suppresses, or overwhelms the body's ability to adapt and maintain healthy function can cause stress. Well-known examples of stress include bereavement, depressive states, and overworking, but cold and damp, poor sleep, and food allergy, as well as positive events such as going on holiday or getting married can all be highly stressful. Much ill health results from routinely pushing the body beyond its limits and failing to recognize the cumulative effect of stress and its impact on mood, vitality, and immune function. Learning your limits can be a painful process but recognizing the signs when you are over-extended means that you have the option to pull back and take action before becoming ill.

Lifestyle changes, complementary treatments such as acupuncture and osteopathy, and appropriate herbal medicines, including tonics and adaptogens, all work best when they are used to prevent illness and maintain healthy function, particularly when this applies to ongoing stress. Tonic herbs make you feel stronger, less tired, and generally more healthy. Adaptogens are plants and mushrooms that aid the body in coping with stress of all kinds, improving stamina and resilience.

+ **Key herbs:** Maca, Korean ginseng, *rhodiola*, ashwagandha

STRESS AND EXHAUSTION

We are all, at different points in our lives, subject to episodes of acute physical and emotional stress. Thankfully, recovery of vitality, health, and well-being normally follows as a matter of course. In contrast, the problem with chronic stress is that it gradually depletes the body's reserves, weakening adrenal gland and nervous system function. Chronic stress raises anxiety levels and over time can cause familiar symptoms such as brain fog, poor memory, and lowered mood, all signs of nervous exhaustion (see p. 89), a state in which you no longer feel fully in control all the time and even minor issues loom larger and appear more threatening than they actually are.

Many health problems follow a similar pattern, with prolonged stress or excess demands weakening or overwhelming a specific system or vital organ. Fatty liver disease and pre-diabetic states both result from long-term stress, leading to a state of exhaustion, respectively in the liver and in the pancreas. Once a state of exhaustion or deficiency is reached, the affected organ has to be rebuilt and new reserves established before it can again function normally.

Appropriate diet, exercise, and relaxation, supplements such as vitamin B complex, and tonic and adaptogenic herbs (see p. 33) will help the body to cope in situations where no let-up is possible. The same approach will aid the body in rebuilding reserves and walking the path back to good health.

+ **Key herbs:** Liquorice and rosemary for adrenal exhaustion; ashwagandha and lemon balm for mental exhaustion; angelica root and maca root for physical exhaustion

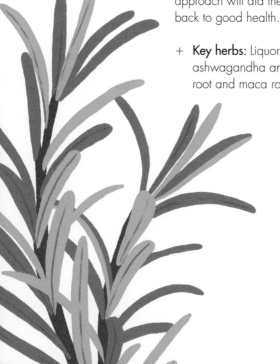

Making Sense of Symptoms

If you wake in the morning after a night out and have a headache, you probably know what caused it and what you need to do about it! Plenty of water, coffee, and a remedy to relieve the headache should help you get on with your day. If you have a headache but did not overdo it the night before, you might wonder why you have a headache, but it is probably safe to ignore for a few hours. But if waking with a headache or developing a headache during the day has become a regular event, this question becomes one that demands an answer.

Minor passing symptoms are a normal part of life, so try not to worry about every passing ache or pain. Too great a focus on the state of your health can become obsessive, and in the long term this will undermine good health. Blocking out symptoms can sometimes be necessary in order to get on with your day, but ignoring persistent symptoms is never a good long-term strategy. Keeping a cool eye on your state of health and using your intelligence to monitor symptoms is generally the best approach. Questioning why you have certain symptoms can bring a clearer picture of what is going on, of your body's strengths and weaknesses, and general patterns of health and ill health.

This section of the book aims to help you make sense of what your body is telling you when you feel unwell, so that with a better understanding you can find and select self-help approaches and herbal remedies that set you on the path back to good health.

NEW SYMPTOMS

New, previously unexperienced symptoms – a sharp pain in the abdomen, for example – can be alarming and it is easy to imagine and fear the worst. Indeed, without reference points or sufficient knowledge, our imagination can run away with us, as can searching online for answers. If symptoms are new and have not occurred before, ask yourself the following questions. Once you have gone through the list, you should have quite a lot of information about your symptom or symptoms. Already, you have some understanding of what is going on. The pages that follow should help you to develop a clearer picture of any health concerns and point you in the direction of effective herbal treatment options.

QUESTIONS
TO ASK

+ **What exactly am I feeling or experiencing right now and has it happened before?**
+ For example: pain, discomfort, disorientation, feeling cold, anxiety, muscle ache.

+ **Can I describe my symptoms? Where are they and what organs or tissues are involved?**
+ For example: indigestion and nausea, eyestrain, sore throat, pain on passing urine.

+ **Is there anything different I have done in the last few days that might be causing this?**
+ For example: a change in diet or different food, anxiety over something or someone, a fall, exposure to infection or pollution.

+ **Is there anything obvious that I can do straight away to help with these symptom(s)?**
+ For example: massage an aching neck, drink some water, go to bed, talk to a friend, take a remedy.

+ **Does anything make my symptoms better or worse, and how long do they go on for?**
+ For example: are they constant, unpredictable, fluctuating, at night only, after meals, when stressed, after exercise?

+ **How severe are these symptom(s)?**
+ If you feel seriously unwell or are in distress, check the list of "red flag" conditions on pp. 22–23 and contact your healthcare practitioner urgently.

RECURRING SYMPTOMS

If you have previously experienced your current symptom(s) – for example, sore throat and raised neck glands or dry and itchy skin – you may very well know what the problem is. You probably also have some idea of how to set about treating it. Even so, taking some time to ask yourself the following questions will help you to fine-tune your response.

+ **Are the symptoms the same as the ones you experienced last time or are there identifiable differences?**
+ For example: have they come back more or less severely or extensively than before in different areas?

+ **Are the symptoms recurring in a shorter (or longer) period of time and with greater (or lesser) frequency?**
+ A shorter gap between symptom outbreaks suggests the problem is getting worse, a longer gap suggests improvement.

+ **What factors may have led to these symptoms coming back again?**
+ If you know that certain factors are responsible, can you do anything to limit their impact?

+ **When you last had these symptoms, what proved to be most helpful in relieving them? Can you repeat this approach and are there other treatment options to explore?**

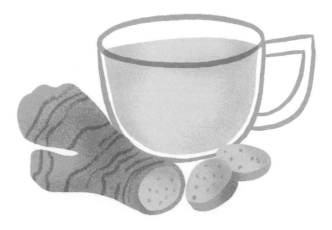

ACUTE SYMPTOMS

Through direct experience, most of us know what an acute symptom is: the sudden onset of food poisoning or influenza is accompanied by acute symptoms that cannot be ignored, a retreat to bed usually being required for several days. Symptoms of acute illness result from a protective response by the body in its attempts to re-establish healthy internal function (homeostasis), for example vomiting and diarrhoea clear out pathogens from the digestive tract, higher body temperatures stimulate immune resistance, helping to counter infectious pathogens.

TRY THIS

+ Rest and relax: This will enable your body to focus on aiding the affected area or organ, or to counter infection.
+ Keep well hydrated: Drinking lots of water aids the body in cleansing.
+ Use herbal remedies: For example, take a ginger infusion or turmeric powder to help control fever, ease pain and discomfort, and counter inflammation.

CHRONIC SYMPTOMS

As the word "chronic" indicates, symptoms may be present for extended periods of time. Chronic ill health typically develops when the body's capacity to repair has been compromised in some way. This can occur after acute illness or emerge after years of niggling, background symptoms. The chronic aches and pains of arthritis and the daily burning pain of acid reflux are examples of situations where cellular self-repair processes, and organ function, are no longer functioning effectively.

TRY THIS

+ Treat your symptoms: In the first instance, take steps to alleviate your symptoms such as ease pain or soothe digestive symptoms. Refer to Chapter 4: Common Ailments for your specific symptom.
+ Support tissue repair: Take herbs that stimulate repair of affected tissues, for example marigold for inflamed skin.
+ Improve the health of underperforming organs. Take herbs that support the specific organ, for example, meadowsweet for acid indigestion and gastritis. Make lifestyle changes that aid this process including, dietary changes, exercise, relaxation, and so on, plus tonic herbs such as ashwagandha.

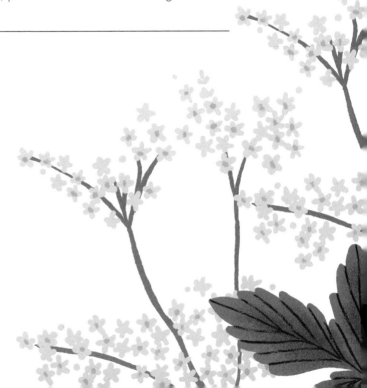

UNDERSTANDING PAIN

Pain is a call for attention to a particular body area or organ. Thinking about what type of pain you have, and what is causing it, can point you towards effective pain relief and treatment. Toothache, for example, is most often caused by local inflammation and infection that causes a dull, throbbing pain around the tooth. If surrounding nerves become affected, pain becomes sharp and more acute and may be felt along the course of a nerve, at sites distant from the inflamed area. Manageable pain levels pain demand pain relief and treatment of the underlying cause(s) – herbal remedies and acupuncture work very well together in this context. If you are experiencing severe or chronic pain (no matter what type) contact your healthcare practitioner. Consult Chapter 4: Common Ailments for specific types of pain.

TYPES OF PAIN AND ASSOCIATED HERBS	
	+ Spasmodic pain, such as in colic and menstrual cramps, results from over-contracted muscles blocking off blood supply and oxygen to the affected tissues.
	+ **Key herbs:** Chamomile, valerian, cramp bark
	+ Inflammatory pain, such as in arthritis and sore throat, results from intense inflammatory activity in the area.
	+ **Key herbs:** Turmeric, echinacea, liquorice
	+ Nerve-based or neuropathic pain, such as in sciatica and shingles, results from nerve irritation, which triggers a pain response.
	+ **Key herbs:** Saffron, Californian poppy, *cannabidiol (CBD)*, St John's wort

HOT AND COLD

In good health, our bodies maintain a stable internal temperature of around 37°C (99°F) and adjust rapidly to temperature change, while in a fever the body works hard to quickly re-establish a normal body temperature. Even when healthy, we sweat to cool down and shiver to generate heat, and we drink cooling or warming drinks depending on the season. Despite this, many of us say we feel too hot or too cold even though our body temperature stays normal.

In herbal medicine, this sense of feeling too hot or too cold is an important factor in understanding what is wrong with a person and deciding what treatment to prescribe. People who feel hot much of the time may have imbalanced or overactive liver, pancreatic, or thyroid function and be irritable and erratic – roughly what is known in traditional Chinese medicine as "liver fire". Conversely, people who feel cold much of the time are likely to have an underactive metabolic rate and thyroid function, as well as poor peripheral circulation, and will often lack energy and decisiveness. The excess heat and flushing that can occur at the menopause is somewhat different, as these symptoms are distinct from the underlying factors affecting the person's sense of heat or cold.

These two extremes are best understood in terms of a spectrum that stretches from hot at one end to cold at the other, with most people sitting somewhere in between, close to average. Thinking where you (or someone you want to help) fit on this spectrum of hot to cold can help in selecting appropriate herbs to "cool" and relax or "warm" and gently stimulate, as required. At the simplest level, someone who is too hot (as in a fever) or who feels hot most of the time, needs cooling and relaxing herbs, such as bitters and digestive remedies, while someone prone to feeling cold needs warming herbs that will increase metabolic rate and strengthen circulation to head, hands, and feet. The aim in each case is to help the body to restore normal function, especially metabolic and circulatory function.

+ **Cooling herbs**
  Artichoke, peppermint, olive leaf, milk thistle, dandelion

+ **Warming herbs** Angelica, Chinese angelica, ginkgo, rosemary, ginger

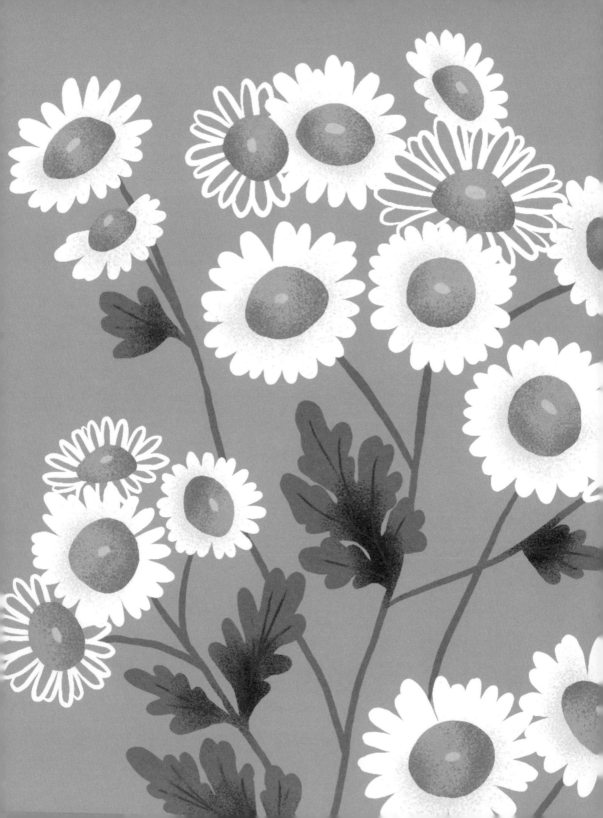

Self-Care and Healing

Looking after yourself is at least as important as any medicine or remedy and can make all the difference in speeding recovery from illness. This chapter makes suggestions about how you can access and use your own resources to recover good health more quickly.

3

What is Good Health?

Self-care and healing play a significant role when it comes to maintaining good health. Medicines of all kinds, including herbal remedies and dietary supplements help to create the conditions in which good health can flourish but they cannot make you actively healthy. This chapter considers what being in "good health" actually means and gives practical advice to help you, or someone in your care, to maintain good health. If you are unwell, this chapter also offers strategies to help you recover more quickly.

ADOPTING A POSITIVE OUTLOOK

Good health is much more than the absence of illness. Having some idea about what good health involves puts you in a better position to assess how well or unwell you are and to consider what steps you might take to improve your state of health physically, mentally, and emotionally.

Good health is dynamic, a state in which your being – body, mind, and soul – is able to function in harmony, without significant inner friction, and to respond positively to life's challenges, be they social, environmental, or emotional, and so on. In this state, both body and mind have reserves to cope with the demands that daily life brings, and though worry and sadness will be present at times, happiness and a positive outlook prevail. The impact of external factors, including concerns that you may have about day-to-day events in the world around you, can make this level of good health seem unattainable. Nevertheless, acting positively to support your health and emotional state at times of difficulty and stress, and appreciating the things that go well in your life, rather than dwelling on those that do not, really does make a difference.

While some people are blessed with good health and experience barely a day's illness, for many, good health comes and goes, and poor health intervenes at different periods in their lives. The pages that follow focus on those areas of your life on which you can focus in order to help you maintain good health and well-being and, hopefully, to shrug off ill health when it threatens to take hold.

A HEALING ENVIRONMENT

A home can be a haven, a place where you can literally let down your hair, shake off the difficulties of the day, unwind, nurture yourself, and let a measure of peace seep into your soul. However, if you have a child who is sick, a moody partner, or a sick parent – to give but a few examples – this picture of home may seem rosy. Yet, it is this ability to nurture yourself, and to care for your own needs at the same time as caring for others, that gives you the best chance of staying healthy if, and when, signs of ill health appear. For most people, home is where self-care has the best chance of flourishing.

A healing environment is a place where emotions can be restored, but it is also any space in which you feel protected and at ease. Making a healing space in your own home, one that other household members respect, can be a boon. It might be in your bedroom or somewhere else where you can just be quiet or mindful or pray, as feels right. Candles and the fragrance of essential oils such as lavender or *ylang ylang* will make the space more your own and uplifting, as will the addition of pot plants, especially herbs.

Learning to recognize places that you visit in your daily life, or find on your travels, that have a healing quality can be a joy. It may be a spot in your garden, a particular tree in a park or woodland, a painting, or a view from a mountainside. Revisiting such healing places can calm the spirit and instil faith that you will find your way through whatever difficulties are besetting you. If you cannot actually go to this place, visualize being there, inspire the air, and feel the sense of peace and well-being that flows around you.

+ See also, Emotional Health (pp. 132–135)

FOOD AND SELF-CARE

Food and nutrition underpin good health and provide the essentials needed to keep well and to maintain healthy function. Food can be one of life's great pleasures. Sharing food with friends and family members is one of the great pleasures in life, infusing a sense of well-being and happiness into all those present. Ideally, we would experience this much of the time, but rushed meals, emotional disagreements, lunchtime meetings, and working late all break the connection between food, good digestion, and social warmth. This may be a reason why cooking for ourselves and eating alone can be so hard. Self-care means feeding yourself with care and attention, and hopefully a modicum of pleasure. If you are alone and find cooking for yourself a challenge, why not invite someone to a meal once or twice a week and cook something special for your guest.

In his book *Food Rules: An Eater's Manual*, Michael Pollan suggests that we should "eat food, not too much, mostly plants". This is a good summary of dietary common sense. Overeating, or eating too much of a specific food such as red meat or ultra-processed foods, has a harmful impact on our health and stimulates inflammatory activity within the body. Routinely eating in an unbalanced way is likely to make you ill in the medium- to long-term. If you are eating excessively, try in the first instance to switch to foods that provide better nutrition – for example, dried fruit in place of biscuits and oat porridge rather than sweetened cereals. These nourishing foods help you to feel full more quickly. There can be an emotional source to overeating – for some, eating can feel like a way to ease emotional pain. Seeking therapeutic support might be the way forward, and also caring consistently for yourself in other ways – by seeing friends more often, making your home a more healing space, or joining a Tai Chi class, for example – are all ways to bring more self-care into your life.

PRESERVING YOUR ENERGY

In our competitive world, we tend to look at others and compare ourselves with them and with how they perform. Comparing ourselves repeatedly to others, instead of affirming our own successes and achievements, is a recipe for losing our sense of self-worth. We are all of us unique and perhaps the biggest challenge in life is to find what we are uniquely good at. Paradoxically, we do not find this uniqueness by trying hard. Rather, knowledge of who we are comes when we allow ourselves to relax into being who we naturally are.

Putting pressure on yourself to compete or to find your place in life leads to over-intensity, a pattern that often results from the desire to be perfect. "Going for broke" is fine when you know that you have found what you really want to put your heart and soul into, but living at this level of intensity all the time, trying to be perfect no matter how trivial the task, is counter-productive. Not only will you find it difficult to unwind and relax, but it is highly inefficient in terms of energy use. By way of example, if you are prone to getting viral infections, a reduced intensity in performing routine tasks at home or work could allow your immune system to strengthen and develop greater resistance to infection.

A pattern of over-intensity and inability to relax can be helped with relaxing exercise such as Pilates, Tai Chi, and yoga. Breathing exercises can be especially helpful. Herbal remedies provide another route in aiding relaxation and reducing pressure to perform.

+ See Anxiety and Stress (p. 134); Irritability and Anger (p. 135)

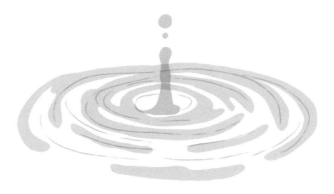

Walking the Path Back to Good Health

Coping with illness – even moderate health problems such as migraine and irritable bowel – can be hard enough on its own, but when it impacts on normal daily life, the consequences can be considerable. The pages that follow aim to provide useful advice that can help you on your way back to good health.

A POSITIVE APPROACH

Keeping positive and focused on the things that will help you to get better is vitally important. One of the reasons why it is good to see a healthcare practitioner is that they can monitor your progress and help keep you focused on the daily things that will help you get well: diet, remedies, medication, relaxation, exercise, and so on. This section is not a substitute for seeing a practitioner, but it may help you in walking the sometimes difficult path back from illness to convalescence to good health.

The 10th-century Persian physician Ibn Sina said that "patience is the beginning of the cure". Having patience and being realistic in your expectations about recovery is extremely important. There are times to push against the boundaries, as in recovery from some sports injuries, but in general when we are ill or unwell, fretting, impatience, and making excessive demands on our bodies, will only slow and delay the process of healing and repair. This is especially true when the body's reserves are low, with little vitality and poor stamina.

DO'S AND DON'TS

+ **DO** seek advice from someone you can trust; a problem shared is a problem halved.

+ **DO** consider whether you are being honest with yourself in assessing your true state of health.

+ **DO** rest and nurture that part of your body that is unwell; give it a breathing space to recover.

+ **DO** trust that you are going to see improvement and recovery but also recognize that this can take time.

+ **DO** be consistent about looking after yourself and taking appropriate herbal remedies and other medication.

+ **DON'T** fall into the trap of repeating unhelpful patterns that may have played a part in you getting ill in the first place, such as going to bed too late, not drinking enough water, and overeating.

+ **DON'T** despair and cast yourself in the role of victim; victims are mostly powerless, whereas patients are not.

+ **DON'T** change a treatment plan that is already underway, unless there are good reasons to do so.

+ **DON'T** undo the recovery that you have made by "running before you can walk".

WHAT TO EAT WHEN ILL

The kitchen is always a good starting place to think about what you can do to help yourself back to better health. If you feel unwell, or are ill, it is wise to avoid foods that will slow down your body's ability to "bounce back" and recover quickly. The following foods are ones best avoided when ill:

+ Sugar, sugar-rich foods and drinks, highly processed foods, fried foods, alcohol; these promote unhealthy bacterial growth in the gut, impair immune function, and stress the liver and pancreas.
+ Mucus-forming foods such as dairy produce and bananas are best avoided, especially in respiratory infections.

Conversely, it makes sense to eat foods that will not burden the body and may actively improve its ability to regain health. Suggestions include:

+ Eating food warm, as much as it is possible
+ Soups and broths with vegetables and chicken
+ Hot drinks with fresh lemon or lime juice, ginger, cinnamon (see The Kitchen Brew p. 103). Note that warm or hot drinks are best in chronic health problems. In fever, hot infusions of herbs such as elderflower will stimulate sweating and lower body temperature, though iced water can also be taken to lower core body temperature
+ Stewed or steamed vegetables, especially carrots, celery, onions, leeks
+ Stewed fruits such as apple, pear, raspberry
+ Fresh fruits such as grapes, blueberries, mango, papaya
+ Oats – in stews, as porridge, or oatcakes
+ Honey, where a sweetener is required

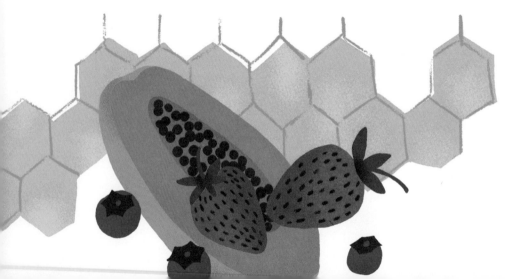

DEALING WITH STRESS AND NEGATIVE EMOTIONS

One of the most difficult aspects of ill health is not knowing how long it will take you to recover so that you can get on with your life again. Planning for the future is difficult, while work, childcare, and keeping up with friends and family may become complicated and stressful. Dealing with stress and the negative emotions that so often accompany ill health – fear and anxiety, anger and depression – are sometimes as challenging as the illness itself.

Everyone's situation is different but there are recognized ways in which you can support yourself, stay positive, and avoid despair. As best you can, stick to dealing with today's concerns, such as getting enough sleep, who is going to shop or cook, and so on. Do not get caught up in "phantom", imaginary problems in the future that may never happen. Negative emotions consume large amounts of nervous energy and leave you in a worse place. Herbal treatment can help with ongoing stress and in relieving negative emotions.

+ See Anxiety and Stress (p. 134); Low Mood (p. 133)

TRY THIS	We only have so many hours in the day, and limited stamina and energy available to you at any given time. Try to use this in as calm and thoughtful a way as possible. Here are some ideas to help you:

+ Learn to recognize when anxiety or depression are getting the upper hand and be willing to ask for help.
+ Allow people to do things for you and, even if they cannot do it as you would like, be appreciative of their efforts.
+ Remember that a tranquil mind and positive outlook will help with your recovery.

BEING KIND TO YOURSELF

As human beings, we are infinitely complex, and trying to tease out the many factors that lie behind ill health can be a near impossible task. Dr Edward Bach wrote that "Behind all disease lie our fears, our anxieties, our greed, our likes and dislikes" (*The Twelve Healers and Other Remedies*, 1930). Whether you agree with this or not, it is clear that emotions are intimately involved in our sense of well-being.

Self-care does not mean being self-indulgent, rather it means giving to yourself the same care and attention that you give to someone you love – a partner, a child, or parent. If your partner is getting frequent headaches or showing signs of depression, you might pick the right moment to ask: What is going on? Why is it happening? What can be done about it?

The same questions apply in terms of self-care. Asking yourself these questions may be painful but there is relief in facing up to difficulties. All too often, we find it hard to be compassionate or kind to ourselves and sometimes this sits strangely at odds with a very real capacity to be kind to others. In our overly competitive world, quietly punishing ourselves for failure, or for doing something wrong, is not unusual, and these thoughts and feelings lie buried within our consciousness, telling us that we are unworthy or useless or do not deserve to be well. Being kind to yourself involves seeing these thoughts for what they are: negative and foolish.

TRY THIS

+ Give more thought to how you can look after yourself and list those things that will help you get better.

+ Allow yourself to be well – be prepared to face those things that are troubling you and move on.

+ Build healing routines into your daily life. Make a smoothie at breakfast, buy healthier food. Take relaxing exercise.

+ Find time each day for yourself to do something creative, spend a while in the garden or in a park, or just being quiet.

+ Give yourself helpful treats (as you might give an unwell friend a treat).

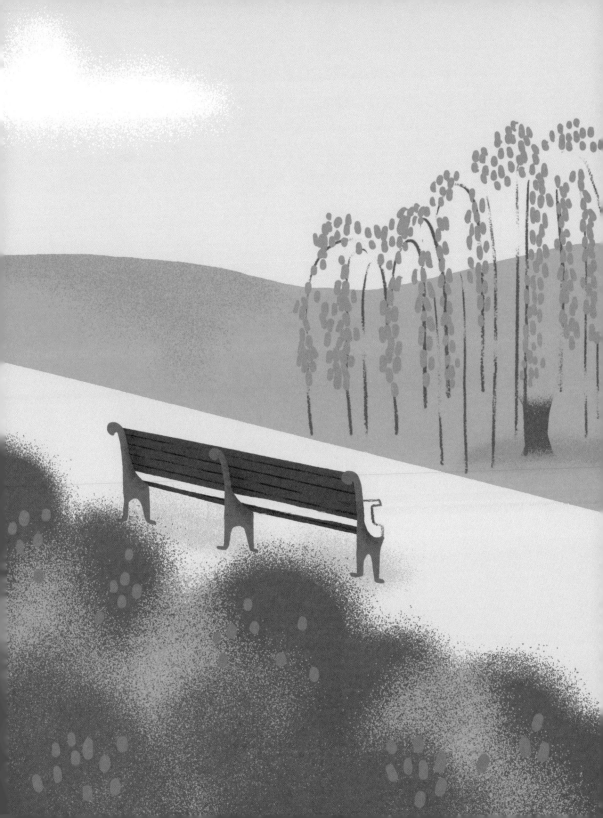

REBUILDING STAMINA AND ENERGY RESERVES

Recovering vitality after long-term illness can be a painfully slow process. The following suggestions focus on the mental self-discipline that enables you to conserve energy as much as possible. The sections on Adaptive Capacity (see p. 33) and Stress and Exhaustion (see p. 34) in Chapter 2: Understanding Health & Illness look briefly at how the body adapts to stress and the effects of chronic stress on vitality and energy reserves. If you have poor vitality or tire easily, these sections are worth re-reading. See Nervous Exhaustion and Tiredness (p. 89) and Low Mood (p. 133) for herbal treatment.

ECONOMIZE

Think in terms of an energy economy: Can you "bank" or "save" energy, build a healthy energy "credit"? Keeping a calm, focused mind minimizes energy loss through anxiety and worry.

ASSESS YOURSELF

Recognize that energy levels fluctuate. Learn to assess your vitality and resilience on a day-to-day basis – a short walk that might be good on one day, but might be too much on another.

CONSERVE ENERGY

Avoid getting overtired. Being overtired can set you back significantly. Learn to use available energy as carefully as possible.

TAKE A REMEDY

Take adaptogen and tonic herbs such as ashwagandha, Korean and Siberian ginseng, maca, rosemary, and thyme.

RECOVER

Recognize that recovery is often three steps forward and two steps back. Look at the medium- to long-term picture.

FIND A ROUTINE

Try and establish a relaxed daily routine that can be slowly extended as energy levels improve. Aim to include toning and relaxing exercises, especially breathing exercises. Eat small frequent nutritious meals.

RETURNING TO NORMAL LIFE

Returning to normal life after a period of illness can be daunting, especially if it has been long-term. Being ill can make you feel that you have entered a separate country from which escape is not straightforward. Not only do you have to walk the path back to good health, but it can feel as if a passport is required to cross the frontier. Nonetheless, if you have reached the point where you are about to resume your normal daily life, with all its demands and responsibilities, you have already come a long way.

The key, perhaps, is to realize that you will not be fully recovered until you are able to complete your daily tasks with the same ease that you did before you became ill. Rather than throwing yourself into frenzied activity to catch up on piles of accumulated work, slowly break yourself back in without overdoing it. Even a week in bed leads to weakened leg muscles that need to be stretched, exercised, and toned, but not overexercised. The same applies to mental activity and work; mental and physical strength and resilience come in large part from practising routines, routines that quietly stretch and tone the mind and body and gradually improve performance.

Adaptogenic and tonic herbs might have been specifically designed to help in this context, supporting the transition back into normal daily life. Such herbs improve stamina and endurance and help to prevent overexhaustion.

+ **Key adaptogen and tonic herbs** Echinacea, maca, Korean ginseng, *goji berries*, rosemary, *rhodiola*, ashwagandha, ginger

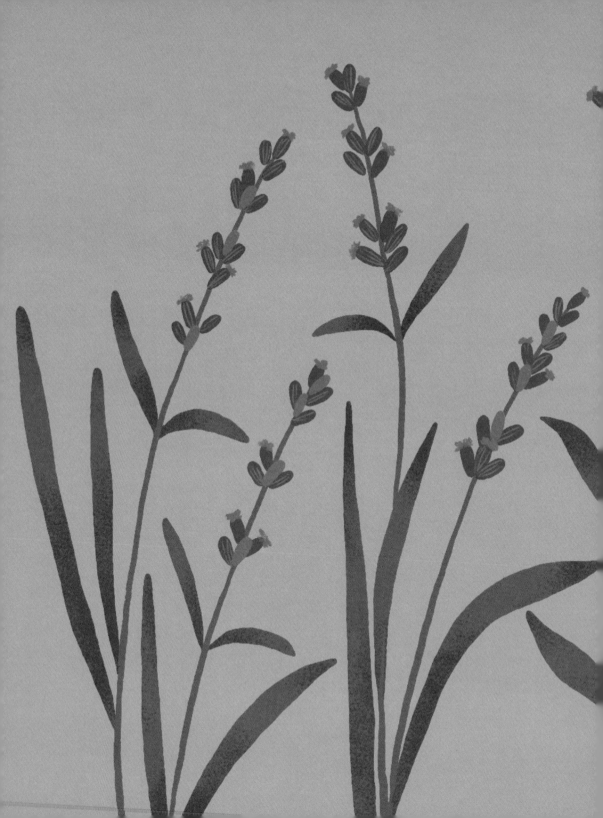

Treating Common Ailments

This chapter provides a comprehensive listing of effective herbal treatments that will help with most common health complaints – from childhood to late adulthood. Wherever possible, there are several treatment options for each ailment, enabling you to choose remedies that closely match your specific health problem.

4

Treating Common Ailments

This chapter offers simple, practical suggestions for healing common health complaints using herbal remedies. It starts with the head and ailments such as headaches, earache, and mouth ulcers, before working its way through the main body systems – muscular, nervous, circulatory, digestive, and urinary. The chapter ends with sections on women's health, men's health, and treating children.

People across the world use thousands of plants as medicines every day, so the treatments recommended in *The Home Herbal* are not exclusive. Neither are they automatically better than other herbal recommendations. Rather, they aim to provide the best possible advice for self-care and treatment using, primarily, the 50 key herbs profiled in Chapter 5. Focusing on just 50 well-known and well-researched herbs means that you have a better chance of becoming familiar with them and, over time, more confident and assured in using them. Where remedies include herbs that do not feature in Chapter 5, these are set in italic. You will find an index of herbs on pages 248–249.

FINDING A REMEDY

There are more than 100 different entries in this chapter, all listed in the index. They cover health problems ranging from everyday illness, such as colds and flu, to long-term problems, such as weight loss, and emotional health issues, such as anger and irritability.

If you have a fall and graze your leg, it is fine simply to look at Cuts, Grazes, and Minor Wounds (p. 71) and decide what treatment is going to work best. You do not need to read the whole book before deciding the best course of action. However, more complex health problems – for example, acid indigestion or severe menstrual cramps – benefit from more thought before you decide how to treat yourself. Look at the entry for your health problem, and then look at the profiles of recommended herbs. If emotions are a major driver behind your symptoms, Chapter 3 may give you a clearer picture of what to do.

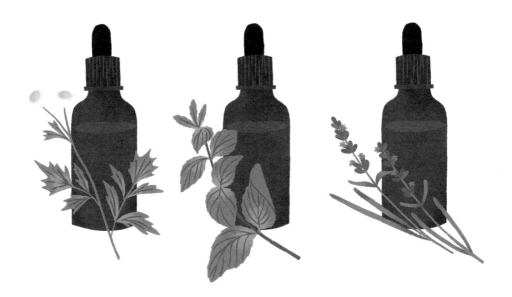

Each remedy comes with suggested ways of taking it, together with appropriate dosages. You are advised to keep to these dosages, as more does not necessarily mean better with herbal medicine. There is, however, no requirement to follow the proposed way of taking the herb – take the recommended herb(s) in whatever form is most suitable for you. Throughout this chapter, where instructions are given for making infusions, simply multiply the dried herb measurement by one and a half if you are using fresh herbs. When concentrated extracts are listed, these are manufactured products that include tablets, capsules, or liquid extracts (see pp. 224–225 for further details on dosage).

Head

Many health problems affect the head, and although they are mostly only troublesome rather than serious, they can have a disproportionate impact on your ability to think clearly and interact with people. The following self-help suggestions aim to bring quick relief to symptoms.

HEADACHE

Many factors can cause headaches and having some idea of what triggers them – poor posture, sinus infection, or dehydration, for example – can help you to select the most appropriate herbs. You can treat an occasional headache symptomatically using some of the herbs suggested below. More regular occurrence of headaches indicates that you may need to make lifestyle changes – adjusting the chair at your workstation, drinking more water, taking time out to eat lunch, and getting more sleep are a few examples.

TREATMENT

+ **General headache** Massage a few drops of lavender or peppermint essential oil, or a "hot" ointment such as *tiger balm*, into the temples or over sore sinuses.
+ **Tension headache** Take a *lime flower* infusion. Make it using 10 g (⅓ oz) dried herb to 200 ml (7 fl oz) water. Take 5 ml (1 tsp) of passion flower or valerian tincture tincture one to three times a day, or take 20 drops of passion flower or valerian tincture an hour, as wanted, or take passion flower or valerian as a concentrated extract. Apply a cold chamomile compress to the forehead.
+ **Poor posture/neck and headache** Massage cramp bark tincture or Healing Oil (see p. 83) into tight muscles.
+ **Sinus congestion** Take a chamomile and/or *eucalyptus* inhalation (see Sinus Problems and Catarrh, p. 105).
+ **For a headache linked to indigestion** Take a peppermint or meadowsweet infusion. Make it using 1–2 teabags to a cup of water or 10 g (⅓ oz) dried herb to 200 ml (7 fl oz) water. Chew 2–5 *cardamom* seeds for 5–10 minutes before spitting out or swallowing, as wanted.

MIGRAINE

The remedies listed for headaches may bring symptomatic relief for a migraine, but the specific herb for migraines is *feverfew*.

TREATMENT

+ Take 5–15 drops of *feverfew* tincture up to five times a day in water or take *feverfew* as a concentrated extract.
+ Eat one small fresh *feverfew* leaf up to three times a day (the old tradition is to eat it in bread).
+ Take ginkgo as a concentrated extract or take 2.5 ml (½ tsp) of gingko tincture one to three times a day. This is best taken long term.

FROM THE GARDEN

+ *Eucalyptus, feverfew,* peppermint

HANGOVER

Drinking plenty of water alongside alcohol intake is one of the best of ways to avoid a hangover. Dehydration causes many of the typical hangover symptoms. The following suggestions will help relieve the symptoms of a hangover.

TREATMENT

+ Make a smoothie with *apple* and *beetroot* and your favourite fruits and vegetables. Add a thumb-sized piece of grated fresh ginger root or 2.5 g (½ tsp) powder, 2.5 g (½ tsp) ground milk thistle seeds (or take milk thistle as a concentrated extract), and a sprig of rosemary. Blend and drink the smoothie slowly.
+ Take a peppermint infusion. Make it using two peppermint teabags to a cup of water or 10 g (⅓ oz) dried herb to 200 ml (7 fl oz) water. Add grated fresh ginger root and lemon juice. This will help with both headache and stomach sensitivity.

FROM THE GARDEN

+ Peppermint, rosemary

DIZZINESS AND LIGHTHEADEDNESS

These might be passing symptoms or can be the side-effects of an underlying health condition. Sometimes low blood pressure and poor circulation to the head are the cause. Contact your healthcare practitioner if dizziness or lightheadedness are frequent problems. (See also, Low Blood Pressure, p. 96).

TREATMENT	+ Massage a few drops of lavender or peppermint essential oil into the temples or behind the ears. + Place 1–5 drops of ginkgo tincture under the tongue or take 20 drops of ginkgo tincture with water up to five times a day, or take gingko as a concentrated extract. + **Where symptoms are linked to emotional stress** Take a lemon balm, *lime flower*, or passion flower infusion. Make it using 10 g (⅓ oz) dried herb to 200 ml (7 fl oz) water and sip it slowly. To increase its strength, add 10 *cardamom* seeds or freshly grated ginger root. + **Where dizziness is linked to fatigue and lowered vitality** Take 2.5 ml (½ tsp) of angelica root, black cohosh, and echinacea tincture, in equal parts, up to five times a day.
FROM THE GARDEN	+ Lemon balm, peppermint

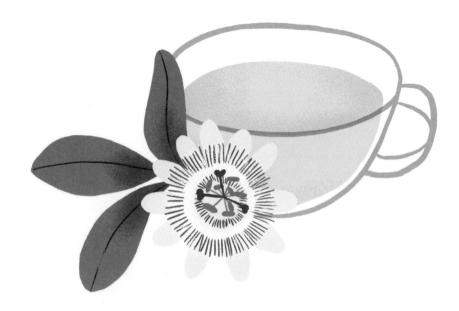

Eyes

The eyes are the most delicate part of our anatomy and need special care and attention. Especially today, with extended hours of screen time, it pays to be alert to signs of eye weakness or overuse.

TIRED OR SORE EYES

Sore or tired eyes are a common sign of overwork. The remedies suggested here should soothe and heal, but resting the eyes more might be the best medicine. If only one eye is affected, do not risk transferring infection to the other one – use separate compresses for each eye.

TREATMENT

+ Make a chamomile infusion using 5 g (2½ tsp) dried herb to 100 ml (3½ fl oz) water or use a warm teabag. Soak cotton wool in the infusion and apply this gently as a compress with the eyelid closed. Allow the infusion to seep into the eye.
+ Soak cotton wool with aloe vera gel, *rose* water, or witch hazel water and apply gently as a compress with the eyelid closed.
+ Drink a marigold and plantain infusion. Make it using 10 g (⅓ oz) dried herb to 200 ml (7 fl oz) water.

FROM THE GARDEN

+ Chamomile, elderflower, plantain

CONJUNCTIVITIS

Use the recommendations as listed in the previous section for topical relief of this common infection. See below for additional remedies.

TREATMENT

+ Consume 10 drops of *eyebright* or propolis tincture in water up to five times a day. Caution: these remedies are both very drying.
+ Consume 20 drops of echinacea and/or thyme tincture up to five times a day, or take either herb as a concentrated extract.

BLEPHARITIS AND STYES

Blepharitis can be a very stubborn condition to treat. As it is a chronic bacterial or fungal infection, cutting back on sugar and alcohol is a good idea, alongside trying the following remedies. Styes will usually clear with these remedies. You may need additional support for the body's immune system.

TREATMENT

+ Cleanse eyelids with aloe vera, applying it as a compress where there is inflammation.
+ Carefully mix 5–10 drops of *goldenseal* tincture in 10 ml (2–3 tsp) of a simple chamomile or marigold cream (not ointment). Apply this sparingly to closed eyelids or a stye twice a day.
+ **To support immune resistance** Take 2.5 ml (½ tsp) of marigold and/or echinacea tincture twice a day, or take marigold and/or echinacea as concentrated extracts.

Ears

The ears generally function well without manifesting problems other than dry or blocked ear canals. Middle ear infection is common in children and you need to treat it effectively. Recurrent ear infections in childhood can lead to chronic ear problems in later life.

TINNITUS

The following herbs are known to be helpful in relieving tinnitus. You should continue treatment for two to three months. However, tinnitus can be very difficult to treat. Where it is becoming a significant problem, it makes sense to see your healthcare practitioner.

TREATMENT

+ Take 2.5 ml (½ tsp) of ginkgo tincture twice a day or take ginkgo as a concentrated extract.
+ Take 20 drops of black cohosh tincture twice a day.
+ Take 20 drops of *feverfew* tincture twice a day.

EARACHE AND INFECTION

Earache can be a distressing problem, more so if it develops into a middle ear infection. Start treatment promptly to allow the selected remedies to control the inflammation and infection, and to prevent it developing into a full-blown infection that requires antibiotic treatment.

<table>
<tr>
<td>TREATMENT</td>
<td>

+ **To help dissolve earwax** Place 1–2 drops of warm olive oil or warm mullein flower oil into the affected ear. See Hot-Infused Oils p. 236.
+ **To relieve pain** Massage 1–3 drops of *geranium* or lavender essential oil on the face and around the outside of the ear (not in it); massage oil into the pinna (the lower fleshy part of the ear).
+ **To treat an infection and stimulate immune resistance** Take a thyme infusion. Make it using 5 g (2½ tsp) dried herb to 200 ml (7 fl oz) water, sweetened with honey. Or take 2.5 ml (½ tsp) of echinacea tincture two to three times a day, or take echinacea as a concentrated extract. Or take 2.5 ml (½ tsp) of echinacea (two parts), marigold (one part), and barberry (one part) tincture two to four times a day. Eat plenty of garlic.

</td>
</tr>
<tr>
<td>FROM THE GARDEN</td>
<td>+ Marigold, echinacea, thyme</td>
</tr>
</table>

GARLIC OIL	As a first-aid measure for earache and infection, you can make garlic-infused oil in just 20 minutes. Crush six garlic cloves and place them in a small, clean pan with 100 ml (3½ fl oz) olive oil. Cover, and simmer as gently as possible on a hob for 15 minutes. Allow the oil to cool, strain it, bottle it, and label the bottle. To use the oil, apply 1–3 drops of warmed garlic oil into the ear canal, let it seep in and plug the ear with cotton wool. Repeat the treatment up to three times a day.

Mouth

The mouth and tongue are highly resilient organs, tasked with many essential functions – secreting, chewing, speech, and breathing among many others. When problems occur, they can be a sign of being run down, and commonly reflect changes in the bacterial population within the mouth.

MOUTH ULCERS AND SORE TONGUE

You can treat the occasional mouth ulcer effectively using a few drops of tincture or essential oil. Frequent mouth ulcers and a sore or ulcerated tongue need more care and consistent treatment that supports tissue healing and promotes a healthier bacterial population within the mouth. Probiotics formulated specifically for the mouth can be helpful and are readily available in pharmacies and online.

TREATMENT	+ **For the occasional mouth ulcer** Dab a drop or two of liquorice or propolis tincture or 1 drop of *clove, myrrh,* or *tea tree* essential oil on the ulcer. All of these will ease discomfort and support healing. Note: Except for liquorice, these remedies will sting on application.
FOR RESISTANT CASES	+ Make a liquorice mouth rinse by adding 20–30 drops of tincture to a glass of water. Swill the tincture in the mouth for 5–10 minutes. + Add 10 ml (2 tsp) of aloe vera gel/juice to a glass of water and swill it in the mouth for 5–10 minutes before swallowing. Add 20–30 drops of *clove,* echinacea, or propolis tincture, as wanted. Repeat up to three times a day. + Take up to 50 ml (3 tbsp) of *sesame* or *coconut* oil and swill it in the mouth for 10 minutes before spitting it out. Repeat this daily.

COLD SORES

Many situations can bring on a cold sore, including exposure to sun, wind, coldness, infection, lowered immune function, and stress. If they occur frequently, this is a sign that the body is run down, with depleted nervous and immune resistance (see also, Nervous Exhaustion, p. 89). You should avoid foods high in arginine, an amino acid found in nuts and seeds such as almonds, peanuts, and coconut, as they are thought to increase the risk of cold sores. The earlier you can catch a cold sore the better – treat it the minute you realize that a cold sore is developing.

TREATMENT

+ Carefully apply ginger juice, which you can extract by placing a chunk of fresh root in a garlic crusher, or juice from fresh lemon balm leaves to the cold sore.
+ Apply lemon balm, propolis, or *thuja* lip salve, cream, tincture, or infused oil, or aloe vera gel or lotion to the cold sore.
+ Apply 1–2 drops of chamomile, *clove*, or *tea tree* essential oil to the cold sore.
+ Drink lemon balm or rosemary tea.
+ **For a recurrent cold sore infection** Take 10–20 drops of propolis tincture three times a day. Or take 2.5 ml (½ tsp) of echinacea tincture once or twice a day or take echinacea as a concentrated extract. Or take a thyme infusion. Make it using 5 g (2½ tsp) dried herb to 200 ml (7 fl oz) water. Or take 2.5 ml (½ tsp) of thyme tincture once or twice a day.

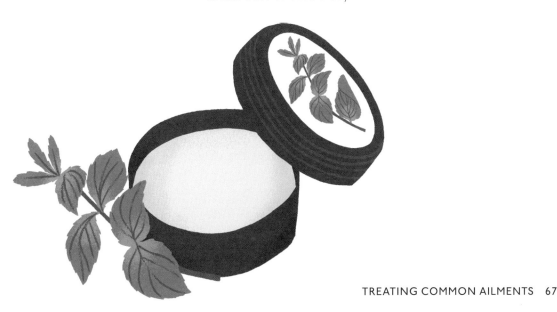

DRY MOUTH

Echinacea stimulates saliva secretion, so is the first remedy to turn to here. Demulcent herbs such as chia seeds provide mucus that will soothe and protect a sore, dry mouth.

TREATMENT

+ Add 25 drops of echinacea tincture to a glass of water and use this as a mouth rinse before swallowing.
+ Combine echinacea tincture (three parts) with liquorice tincture (one part) and take 25 drops up to five times a day.
+ Soak chia seeds in water for 30 minutes until a jelly forms. Swill the jelly, complete with seeds, around mouth before swallowing.

BLEEDING GUMS

Bleeding gums indicate a need for better dental hygiene and bacterial balance within the mouth. Oral probiotics may help.

TREATMENT

+ Make a sage infusion using 10 g (⅓ oz) fresh or 5 g (2½ tsp) dried herb to 200 ml (7 fl oz) water. Brew the infusion for 15 minutes and use it as a mouth rinse.
+ Dab marigold tincture onto a bleeding gum; this will sting.
+ **To help strengthen spongy gums** Take a *yarrow* infusion. Make it using 5 g (2½ tsp) dried herb to 200 ml (7 fl oz) water. Take 2.5 ml (½ tsp) *yarrow* tincture once a day. In either case rinse mouth well and swallow.
+ Take *bilberry*, *grapeseed*, and/or *green tea* as concentrated extracts.

BAD BREATH

Herbs have been used for thousands of years to sweeten the breath.

TREATMENT

+ **To freshen the breath** Chew a few *cardamom* seeds, *coriander* seeds, fennel seeds, fresh *parsley* leaves, or fresh peppermint leaves for 5–10 minutes. Swallow them or spit them out, as wanted.
+ **To sweeten the breath** Swill the mouth with 10 drops of liquorice tincture diluted in a little water up to four times a day.
+ **Bad breath caused by tooth and gum problems** Gargle with 10 drops of propolis tincture diluted in a glass of water.

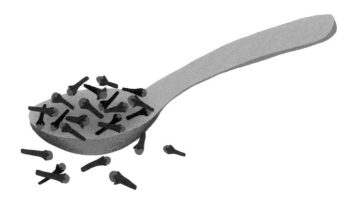

TOOTHACHE

The following are helpful first-aid remedies but are not an alternative to dental treatment.

GENERAL FIRST AID

+ **To ease pain** Apply 1–2 drops of neat clove oil to the site or chew a dried clove. This remedy is also antibacterial.
+ **If you have lost a filling** Cleanse the tooth. Mix clove oil with *marshmallow* root or *slippery elm* powder until it forms a puttylike consistency and use this to plug the hole. You can use peppermint oil in place of clove oil.
+ **To counter inflammation and help relieve pain** Take turmeric as a concentrated extract. (See also, Nerve Pain, p. 92)
+ **To soothe inflammation and help relieve pain in the case of toothache or an abscess** Apply a compress soaked in a warm chamomile infusion to the cheek overlying the site. Make the infusion using 10 g (⅓ oz) dried herb or a teabag to 200 ml (7 fl oz) water. Massage a few drops of lavender oil on the skin overlying the site.
+ Hold an echinacea tablet in place next to the site of infection until it dissolves; this can mildly burn the gum.

Skin

Our skin reflects the general state of our health and can change in appearance and tone from one day to the next. Reading what our skin is telling us can be a useful guide in assessing ill health. The skin and the nervous system develop from the same tissue in the foetus, so it is not fanciful to recognize that our skin gives some indication of our nervous and emotional state – chronic stress, emotional distress, and significant illness remove the bloom of good health normally found in the skin. You can resolve most minor skin problems quickly with antiseptic and wound-healing remedies but more stubborn or serious skin problems will usually need additional internal treatment. This includes making dietary changes (usually the best option is to follow a Mediterranean-type diet), and taking nutritional supplements, such as omega-3 oils and probiotics, and internal herbal remedies such as marigold, echinacea, and turmeric.

BRUISES AND SPRAINS

Although bruising typically spreads for the first few days following an impact, herbs are highly effective in speeding up tissue healing. Arnica is a key remedy for bruising and brings pain relief. The following advice is equally useful following accidents and operations.

GENERAL FIRST AID	+ Chop or mash comfrey or plantain leaves (either fresh or infused dried leaves) and rub or bandage them onto the affected area. + Apply arnica lotion, cream, or ointment two to three times a day.
ADDITIONAL MEASURES	+ **To relieve pain** Massage neat lavender oil into the affected area. + **Where there is a sprain as well as bruising** Apply comfrey oil, cream, or ointment. + **Where there is extensive bruising** Take aloe vera gel or juice internally to encourage systemic healing.

SCARS

Scars form where damaged skin is unable to recover the elasticity of healthy skin. Herbs that promote tissue healing may enable scar tissue to heal more effectively.

TREATMENT

+ Apply aloe vera gel or lotion to the scar twice a day, treating new or recent scars for one to three months and long-standing scars for up to six months. Marigold and comfrey ointment offer good alternatives.

CUTS, GRAZES, AND MINOR WOUNDS

Herbal medicine is generally safe for all but serious wounds and will promote healing and reduce the risk of scarring.

GENERAL FIRST AID

Carefully wash out any grit or glass until the wound is clean. Press firmly on the wound to stem bleeding and maintain pressure for one to two minutes. Cleanse the area well, using aloe vera gel. You can also use a marigold infusion. Make it using 5 g (2½ tsp) dried herb to 200 ml (7 fl oz) boiling water. Alternatively use 25 ml (1½ tbsp) of marigold or echinacea tincture diluted in 200 ml (7 fl oz) boiled water. Firmly apply a clean lint-free cloth (or cotton wool) soaked in witch hazel water or aloe vera gel as a compress over the cut.

ADDITIONAL
MEASURES

+ **To prevent and treat infection or to relieve pain** Apply 1–2 drops of lavender, thyme, or *tea tree* essential oil directly to the wound. Bathe the wound regularly with diluted echinacea tincture or apply mashed garlic with a dressing that you change daily. Seek medical advice if there is no improvement after three days.
+ **To control inflammation and promote tissue repair** Apply marigold, chamomile, or plantain cream or ointment directly to the site of the wound. Apply a plaster or bandage as required. This will also promote tissue repair.
+ **To treat a wound that becomes infected** Bathe it regularly with diluted echinacea tincture or apply mashed garlic with a dressing that you change daily. Seek medical advice if there is no improvement after three days.

BURNS AND SUNBURN

Burns and sunburn respond well to herbal remedies and several herbs even protect against sunburn when taken internally, notably Korean ginseng, lemon balm, and rosemary. You must seek treatment from a healthcare practitioner or hospital for all large burns and those that cause charred skin or significant blistering.

GENERAL FIRST AID

+ Hold the burn under a cold running tap for 20 minutes. Apply aloe vera or simple herbal creams to small burns. On larger areas, apply aloe vera gel or juice across the whole area, keeping it cool for several hours to lessen pain and inflammatory damage. Honey is also effective in place of aloe vera. Bandage small, deep burns with a lint-free cloth that you have bathed in aloe vera gel or juice, or witch hazel water.

ADDITIONAL MEASURES

+ If aloe vera gel, honey, and witch hazel water are unavailable, use cold *green* or *black tea*.
+ **Small burns and sunburn** Apply neat lavender essential oil to soothe the initial pain.
+ **Long-term pain** Apply chamomile cream or aloe vera gel mixed with 4–10 drops of lavender or peppermint oil per 10 ml (2 tsp) cream/gel.
+ Taken internally as concentrated extracts, *boswellia* or turmeric will counter inflammation of the skin and help relieve pain. This is particularly useful in severe cases of sunburn.

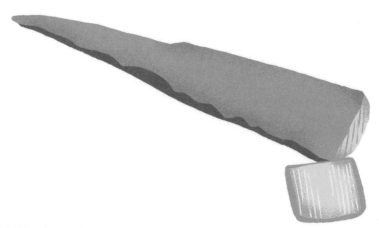

ACNE AND BOILS

Topical herbal remedies will speed the healing of acne while improving the skin's resistance to local infection. Internal treatment to further strengthen skin resistance and promote elimination is often necessary. Self-help measures can often be extremely helpful, but acne can be a stubborn problem requiring professional advice and treatment. Recurring outbreaks of boils can be a sign of diabetes. Skin-brushing and toning help to improve skin resistance. A suitable diet – that is, one low in sugar and dairy produce – supplements including probiotics, and reduced stress levels, all help.

TREATMENT

+ Taken internally, as an infusion and in equal parts, marigold, echinacea, and *red clover* make a good combination for acne. Make the infusion using 10 g (⅓ oz) dried herb to 200 ml (7 fl oz) water. Chaste berry tincture (20 drops a day) can also help in lowering excess testosterone levels.
+ **To control inflammation and promote healing** Apply chamomile or marigold cream routinely to spots. Add *geranium* or *tea tree* essential oil at 10 drops per 10 ml (2 tsp) cream. Apply 1 drop of *geranium* or *tea tree* essential oil directly to the acne spot head (do not burst).
+ **To encourage quicker healing and prevent scar formation** Apply aloe vera gel or lotion or comfrey cream.
+ **To tighten and tone the skin** Apply witch hazel water to greasy areas of the face and spots after washing.
+ Neat *sea buckthorn* and *evening primrose* oils can be helpful in strengthening skin immune resistance and preventing scarring. Test first, then apply sparingly once a day to affected areas.

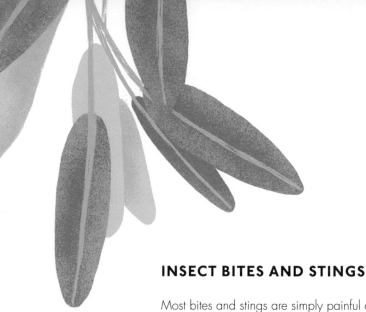

INSECT BITES AND STINGS

Most bites and stings are simply painful and unpleasant, but serious allergic reactions do sometimes occur and require urgent medical treatment. Natural insect repellents include *citronella*, *eucalyptus*, and lavender essential oils, which are especially good against midges.

GENERAL FIRST AID

+ Apply neat lavender essential oil frequently to the painful area. Peppermint, *geranium*, and *clove* essential oils are also good. Use 1–2 drops on small areas or dilute 10 drops to 10 ml (2 tsp) cream. These are all strongly antiseptic and will help relieve pain and inflammation.
+ **Inflammation and swelling** Apply aloe vera gel, a marigold infusion or a chamomile infusion. Make the infusion using 10 g (⅓ oz) dried herb to 200 ml (7 fl oz) water. Apply witch hazel water as a compress. Apply chamomile tincture (dilute in water) as a skin wash and take it internally to soothe and counter inflammation.
+ **Wasp and bee stings** Neutralize wasp stings with vinegar and bee stings with bicarbonate of soda. Apply either as a compress on the site of the sting.

ADDITIONAL MEASURES

+ Chop or mash fresh sage leaves and hold or bandage them on the bite or sting.

FROM THE GARDEN

+ Marigold, chamomile, sage

ITCHINESS, ALLERGIC RASHES, AND ECZEMA

Environmental factors, such as pollen and pollution, and internal inflammatory processes can all cause itchiness. As far as possible, avoid scratching itchy areas as this weakens the skin and creates a risk of infection. Keep yourself well hydrated and the itchy area moisturized. Dry, itchy skin needs "feeding" – applying neat *evening primrose* oil can be helpful. Topical treatment may be sufficient to soothe itchiness and irritation. There is no one go-to remedy, so experiment and find ones that work for you. Sometimes, rotating between different herbs and products works best. Always test a small area of skin first, when applying something new. Internal treatment is often required too.

EXTERNAL TREATMENT	+ **To soothe itchiness and reduce inflammation and irritation** Apply a chamomile, marigold, or *chickweed* infusion or cream. Add 4 drops of peppermint essential oil to 10 ml (2 tsp) cream to reduce itchiness and to cool. Add 10 drops of liquorice tincture to 10 ml (2 tsp) cream to ease chronic itching and allergic rashes. + **Weeping itchy skin and allergic rashes** Apply aloe vera gel/juice or witch hazel water. Note: these can be too drying. + **Itchy fungal conditions especially on the scalp** Sparingly apply *apple cider vinegar*, diluted with water.
INTERNAL TREATMENT	+ **To soothe itchy and allergic skin conditions** Take a chamomile and/or nettle infusion. Make it using 10 g (⅓ oz) dried herb to 200 ml (7 fl oz) water. + Take 20 drops of liquorice tincture up to three times a day and 25 ml (1½ tbsp) aloe vera juice once a day.
FROM THE GARDEN	+ Marigold, chamomile, nettle leaf

FUNGAL SKIN INFECTION

Healthy skin keeps bacteria and fungi on the body's surface under balanced control. Fungal overgrowth causes fungal infections, such as athlete's foot and candida, indicating that the skin's immune resistance has been compromised. The best course of action is to treat the fungal infection while simultaneously supporting skin health.

EXTERNAL TREATMENT

+ Marigold cream, chamomile cream, and *coconut* oil all have antifungal activity and promote skin healing. Add 5–10 drops of *geranium*, thyme, or *tea tree* essential oil to 10 ml (2 tsp) cream to strengthen their effectiveness.
+ **Athlete's foot or fungal nail infections** Apply a few drops of neat *geranium*, thyme, or *tea tree* essential oil.
+ **Vulval and crural (jock itch) fungal infections** Apply chamomile cream mixed with 5 drops of *geranium* oil per 10 ml (2 tsp) cream.
+ **Itchy fungal rashes and dandruff** Apply aloe vera gel/juice or *apple cider vinegar* (neat or diluted).
+ **Chronic fungal skin problems** Apply a *pau d'arco* decoction to the skin. Make it by simmering 10 g (⅓ oz) dried herb in 300 ml (10½ fl oz) water for 15 minutes. Strain the liquid, allow it to cool, and use it as a skin wash.

INTERNAL TREATMENT

+ **To cleanse and support skin health** Take a marigold and *red clover* infusion. Make it using 10 g (⅓ oz) dried herb to 200 ml (7 fl oz) water.
+ **Chronic fungal problems** Take 5 ml (1 tsp) of echinacea, marigold, and *pau d'arco* tincture (equal parts) twice a day.
+ Increase garlic, ginger, and turmeric intake in your diet and take turmeric as a concentrated extract.

WARTS AND VERRUCAS

Apply one of the following remedy choices once a day and cover the
wart or verruca with a plaster or tape after applying the herb. For the
best results, continue treatment for several weeks or months.

TREATMENT

+ Gently massage 1–3 drops of *thuja* tincture into the area.
+ Apply 1 drop of *tea tree, thuja,* or *lemon* essential oil to the site.
+ Gently rub a small mashed garlic clove into the area.

Hair

Poor hair growth or loss may be linked to nutritional deficiency (especially iron), hormonal imbalance, and poor blood flow to the head and scalp. Herbal remedies can provide gentle support and nourishment for the hair, improving scalp health and hair growth.

COMMON PROBLEMS

EXTERNAL
TREATMENT

+ **To promote hair growth, strengthen brittle hair, and to treat dandruff** Make a paste by mixing 20 g (¾ oz) neutral henna powder with water and massage the paste into the scalp and hair. Test the paste for colour first. Apply the paste at night and wash it out in the morning. Repeat every one to three weeks, as needed.
+ **To tone and stimulate hair growth, improve highlights in blonde hair, and to treat dandruff** After washing, rinse the hair with a chamomile and/or marigold infusion. Make it using 10 g (⅓ oz) dried herb to 300 ml (10½ fl oz) water. This is suitable for young children.
+ **To improve circulation to the scalp and darken hair** After washing, rinse the hair with a rosemary, nettle and/or sage infusion. Make it using 10 g (⅓ oz) dried herb to 300 ml (10½ fl oz) water.
+ **Poor hair and scalp health** Add 1–2 drops of chamomile, rosemary, sage, or thyme essential oil to conditioner and wash it out as usual.
+ **Dandruff** Olive oil, *coconut* oil, and *apple cider vinegar* all nourish the hair and scalp and are effective treatments. For the best results, apply the oil at night and wash it out in the morning.
+ **Hair loss** Take a thyme infusion. Make it using 5 g (2½ tsp) dried herb to 200 ml (7 fl oz) water. Take 2.5 ml (½ tsp) of thyme tincture once or twice a day. Massage a thyme infusion or diluted thyme tincture into the scalp on a routine basis.
+ **Receding hair and balding (men and women)** Take saw palmetto as a concentrated extract for at least three months.

FROM THE GARDEN

+ Nettle leaf, rosemary, sage, and thyme

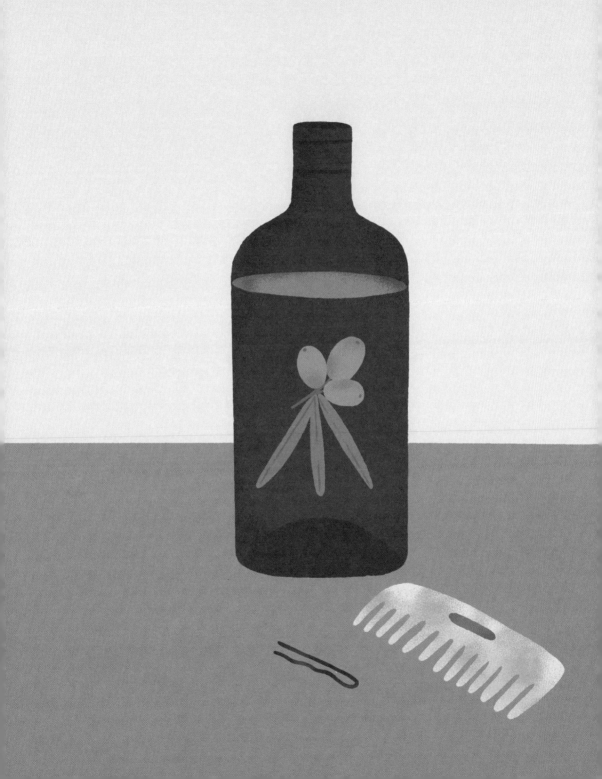

Your Immune System

Our immune systems are immensely complex and intimately connected with our overall state of health. Though infections can, and do, take root, despite good health and a vital immune response, viral and bacterial infections typically occur when the body's reserves are low and immune function is depressed. The question arises: What is causing the infection – a "seed" (virus or bacteria) or the "soil" (the state of our internal environment)?

Both are involved, but examples throughout the natural world suggest that the soil is the key factor. Some plants produce more than 100,000 seeds, yet none of these seeds will manage to germinate where soil and environmental conditions are hostile. The same is true with respect to our soil, the "psycho-neuro-immune" system – our combined ability to respond to challenges of all kinds, including those posed by pathogens, such as viruses and bacteria. A healthy immune system and internal environment usually see off such challenges.

Some people never get ill and are blessed with strong, healthy immune systems. Many people, however, have immune systems that vary in strength and weaken at times of stress, making them prone to recurrent infections. Herbs can be especially valuable in this context, helping to reduce the impact of stress on the body and strengthening immune resistance. Where the body's response to infection is only partly effective and becomes compromised, chronic illness and chronic fatigue can set in. While there are no instant effective treatments for these problems, herbal medicine has much to offer in treating chronic infection and fatigue and steady improvement can, and does, occur.

GENERAL TREATMENT

+ For antiviral, immune support take barberry, echinacea, garlic, liquorice, olive leaf, propolis, and thyme.
+ As adaptogens, take ashwagandha, Korean ginseng, liquorice, maca, and *rhodiola*.
+ Anti-inflammatory herbs such as chamomile, ginger, rosemary, and turmeric can also prove valuable, as can supplements including *bilberry, grapeseed,* or *green tea*.
+ Herbs for the liver – dandelion and milk thistle – may also be needed.

Read up on these herbs, note the recommended doses, and select the ones that are the best fit for you, are affordable, and convenient to take. You will need to be comfortable with taking them long-term. Start with a low dose and slowly increase it. A good plan is to combine the following:

+ At least two antiviral/immune herbs
+ One or more adaptogens
+ One or more anti-inflammatory herbs

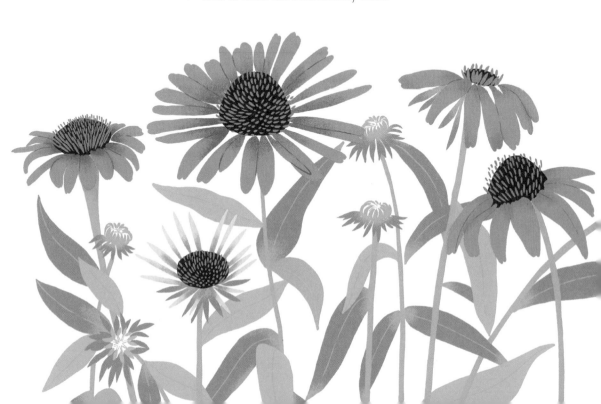

Joints, Muscles, and Bones

Connective tissue, such as muscle, cartilage, and bone, depends on effective circulation to stay healthy. Poor circulation means poor delivery of nutrients and poor removal of waste products. In turn, this leads to slower tissue repair and an increased probability of inflammation. Taking anti-inflammatory remedies, such as turmeric and *boswellia*, will counter inflammation, but the aim should be to prevent underlying inflammation and improve circulation – with appropriate exercise (such as yoga and Tai Chi), circulatory tonics such as *chilli*, gingko, and *yarrow*, and herbs that promote tissue healing, such as comfrey and *gotu kola*.

GENERAL TREATMENT

+ **To encourage tissue repair** Apply comfrey or plantain oil or cream, or neat lavender essential oil to the painful area.
+ Massage Healing Oil (see box) into sore and stiff areas up to five times a day.

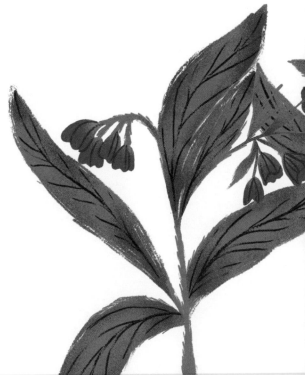

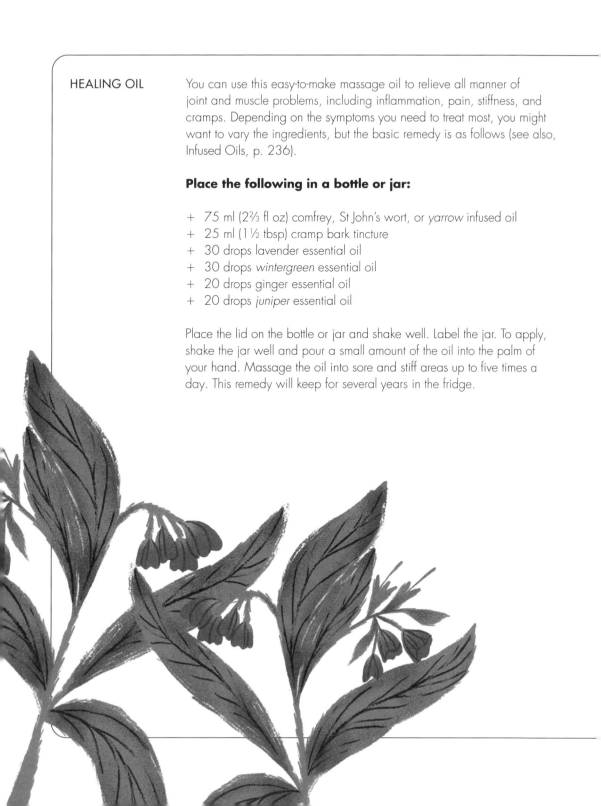

HEALING OIL

You can use this easy-to-make massage oil to relieve all manner of joint and muscle problems, including inflammation, pain, stiffness, and cramps. Depending on the symptoms you need to treat most, you might want to vary the ingredients, but the basic remedy is as follows (see also, Infused Oils, p. 236).

Place the following in a bottle or jar:

+ 75 ml (2⅔ fl oz) comfrey, St John's wort, or *yarrow* infused oil
+ 25 ml (1½ tbsp) cramp bark tincture
+ 30 drops lavender essential oil
+ 30 drops *wintergreen* essential oil
+ 20 drops ginger essential oil
+ 20 drops *juniper* essential oil

Place the lid on the bottle or jar and shake well. Label the jar. To apply, shake the jar well and pour a small amount of the oil into the palm of your hand. Massage the oil into sore and stiff areas up to five times a day. This remedy will keep for several years in the fridge.

CHRONIC JOINT PAIN AND STIFFNESS

Often having taken many years to develop and cause noticeable symptoms, chronic arthritis usually needs patient, ongoing treatment. If the joint is still intact, full recovery is possible but a realistic aim is to improve joint function and minimize pain and discomfort. If the affected joints are weight-bearing, it can be helpful to lose weight, see p. 123.

TREATMENT

+ Massage Healing Oil (see p. 83) into the affected area two to four times a day.
+ Take *boswellia*, turmeric, or *willow bark* as concentrated extracts.
+ Take 5 ml (1 tsp) of cramp bark, *gotu kola*, and nettle tincture in equal parts two to four times a day.
+ Make a foot or hand bath using horsetail, meadowsweet, nettle, rosemary, and/or *yarrow*. See Infusions and Decoctions (pp. 232–233) for preparing this. Or add an infusion to a full-size bath.
+ Add 300 g (10½ oz) Epsom salts (magnesium sulphate) to a warm bath and soak for 15 minutes. This can be very soothing. It will ease joint discomfort and aid sleep.
+ **Inflammatory arthritis, including rheumatoid arthritis** Take *devil's claw* as a concentrated extract.

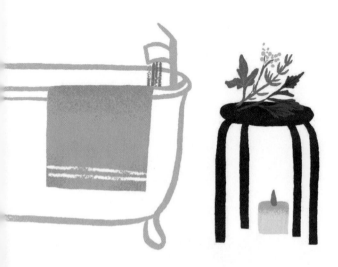

ACUTE JOINT INFLAMMATION AND GOUT

Sudden inflammatory joint pain and gout can be severe. It is best to treat both vigorously with anti-inflammatories and herbs that promote the clearance of waste products, such as urates (the salts in uric acid).

+ **Inflammation and pain** Take *boswellia* or turmeric as concentrated extracts. Take a meadowsweet infusion. Make it using 10 g (⅓ oz) dried herb to 200 ml (7 fl oz) water.
+ **Acute flare-up** Take 5 ml (1 tsp) of *celery* seed (one part), nettle (two parts), and *willow bark* (two parts) tincture three to five times a day and reduce the dose over time. Drink fresh *celery* and *carrot* juice and lots of water.
+ **Pain and tension** Take 20–30 drops of valerian tincture up to six times a day or take valerian as a concentrated extract.

FROM THE GARDEN

+ Nettle, rosemary, *yarrow*

BACKACHE, MUSCLE PAIN, AND CRAMPS

Backache is common and often difficult to treat. Apply Healing Oil (see p. 83) or neat cramp bark tincture to relax tense muscles and ease inflammation. Where muscle tension is the main problem, see cramps. Posture is important: gently open up the chest and lift the ribcage, breathing in deeply. Backache can also be due to referred pain or inflammation from within the abdomen or pelvis – diverticular disease, for example. If this is the case, you need to treat the underlying problem.

TREATMENT

+ **Tense muscles** Massage in Healing Oil, a few drops of lavender essential oil, or a "hot" oil such as *tiger balm*.
+ **Backache and muscle pain** Take *boswellia*, turmeric, or *willow bark* as concentrated extracts.
+ **Cramps** Take 5 ml (1 tsp) of cramp bark tincture up to five times a day (for short-term use). Take 5 ml (1 tsp) of cramp bark and chamomile tincture in equal parts, three times a day, as wanted. Massage cramp bark tincture (or decoction) or horse chestnut gel/cream into cramping muscles. Chronic cramping may indicate a magnesium deficiency.

WEAK MUSCLES

Several herbs are thought to improve muscle strength and tone, particularly after chronic illness. Weak muscles may also result from hypermobility. Supplementing with *bilberry, grapeseed, green tea*, or resveratrol extracts will support collagen formation. Regular toning and exercise will help alongside the remedies.

TREATMENT

+ **To promote muscle fibre and reduce fatty tissue** Take 5–10 g (1–2 tsp) of ashwagandha powder a day or take ashwagandha and Korean ginseng as concentrated extracts.
+ **To support tissue repair after physical trauma, especially nerve tissue** Take 1–2 g (up to ½ tsp) of *gotu kola* powder or 2.5–5 ml (½–1 tsp) of *gotu kola* tincture, daily.
+ For a remedy with general anabolic activity, take 2.5–7.5 g (½–1½ tsp) of maca powder, daily.

FRACTURES AND BROKEN BONES

In the case of fractures and broken bones, topical herbal treatment will often significantly increase the rate of healing and support effective repair of damaged tissue. In situations where healing is slow or incomplete, internal remedies will also be useful. Do not apply remedies to broken bones until they have been correctly re-set – for example, having been in a cast. See also, Bruises and Sprains, p. 70.

TREATMENT

+ For topical applications, use aloe vera gel, juice, or cream, comfrey ointment or plantain ointment.
+ **For internal remedies promoting effective tissue repair** Take up to 6 g (1–1½ tsp) of ashwagandha powder a day or take ashwagandha as a concentrated extract. Or take 2.5 ml (½ tsp) of *gotu kola* tincture one to three times a day. Or take a daily plantain infusion. Make it using 10 g (⅓ oz) dried herb to 200 ml (7 fl oz) water. Or take 2.5 ml (½ tsp) of *yarrow* tincture once a day.

FROM THE GARDEN

+ Comfrey, plantain, *yarrow*

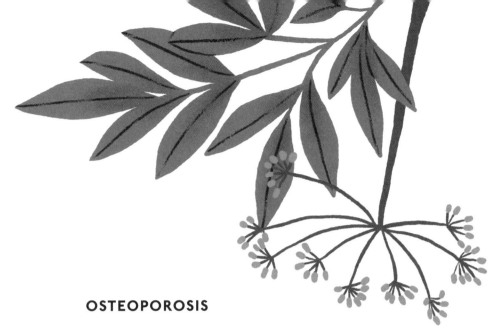

OSTEOPOROSIS

Osteoporosis, and the earlier stage of osteopenia, result, at least in part, from chronic inflammation within the body, which slows down the reformation of bone tissue. Oestrogen has a protective activity against osteoporosis and is strongly anti-inflammatory, so in women osteoporosis tends to be an issue from the time of the menopause onwards. Osteoporosis is less common in men but becomes more prevalent with age. Controlling inflammation and supporting hormonal balance helps to slow or prevent osteoporosis, and early-stage research studies point to several herbs having the potential to help when they are taken long-term at low dosages.

TREATMENT	+ For a hormonal tonic, take 20–30 drops of black cohosh tincture a day. Or take two to three fresh sage leaves or 20–30 drops of sage tincture a day. Or take 2.5 ml (½ tsp) of Chinese angelica tincture once or twice a day. + **To support tissue repair and bone reformation** Take 5 ml (1 tsp) of *gotu kola* and horsetail tincture in equal parts twice a day. Taking 6 g (1 tsp) of ashwagandha powder a day or taking ashwagandha as a concentrated extract is also beneficial. + As an anti-inflammatory, take turmeric powder or take turmeric as a concentrated extract.
FROM THE GARDEN	+ Sage

Nervous System

A healthy, functioning nervous system is the basis of good health and the place where physical, mental, and emotional well-being intertwine. Each of these three affects the others – physical illness has consequences for mental and emotional health, and so on. Thinking about the involvement of the nervous system in any chronic health problem is always worthwhile, particularly as the vagus nerve – the nerve that innervates the heart, lungs, liver, and gut – is frequently involved in apparently physical problems such as acid reflux, irritable bowel, obesity, and weight gain.

Given the limited scope of this book, only the most straightforward problems affecting nervous and emotional health are covered here. The role of herbs in providing gentle supportive treatment to stabilize and strengthen central nervous system function should not be underestimated. Lemon balm, rosemary, and sage are all thought to enhance cognitive function and prevent or slow progression of dementia, while St John's wort is known to act on at least five different neuronal pathways linked to low mood and depression, illustrating the subtle, complex ways in which herbs work.

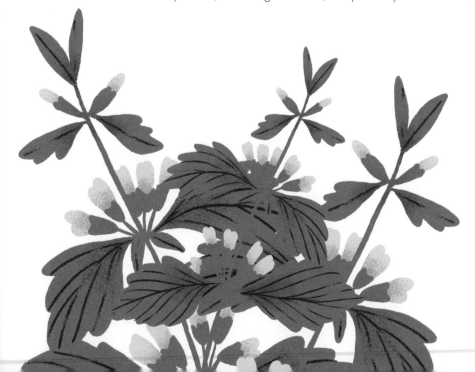

NERVOUS EXHAUSTION AND TIREDNESS

Nervous exhaustion is typically linked to overwork, chronic stress, and inadequate sleep, where the body's ability to recover and repair from excess demands has been compromised. Taking herbal tonics to support the central nervous system and adrenal glands makes good sense. It can be hard to work out whether you are simply exhausted or in fact have chronic fatigue (see Your Immune System, pp. 80–81). As a rule, people with nervous exhaustion, but not chronic fatigue, feel better with gentle exercise, such as relaxed walking, Tai Chi, or yoga. Gentle exercise and mindfulness – keeping focused on positive things and away from worries and stressful demands – are key factors in recovering health after a period of nervous exhaustion.

TREATMENT

+ **To relieve anxiety and stress, encourage relaxation, and improve sleep quality** Take 5 ml (1 tsp) of lavender, lemon balm, valerian, or passion flower tincture once or twice a day. Or take St John's wort as a concentrated extract. These remedies will encourage relaxation and improve sleep quality.
+ **To support better vitality** Take 1 ml (¼ tsp) of liquorice tincture twice a day and 2.5 ml (1 tsp) of rosemary tincture twice a day. Both are key adrenal tonics.
+ **To promote stamina and nervous reserves** Take up to 6 g (1 tsp) of ashwagandha powder a day or take ashwagandha, Korean ginseng, or *rhodiola* as concentrated extracts.
+ *Goji berry*, maca powder, *oats*, and saffron are also beneficial.

A COMBINATION
OF REMEDIES
FOR NERVOUS
EXHAUSTION

+ Take lemon balm and passion flower in equal parts, either as an infusion that you make using 10 g (⅓ oz) dried herb to 200 ml (7 fl oz) water, or as 5 ml (1 tsp) of combined tincture that you take one to three times a day.
+ Take 20 drops of liquorice tincture twice a day.
+ Take *rhodiola* as a concentrated extract.
+ Consume a handful of *goji berries* a day, 10 strands of saffron a day, and up to 5 g (1 tsp) of maca powder a day.

POOR MEMORY AND CONCENTRATION

Research shows that many medicinal plants support healthy brain function, encouraging better circulation within the central nervous system, countering inflammatory processes, and aiding nerve cell regrowth and repair. Key herbs that enhance memory and cognition are listed below. Good hydration and a healthy, mostly vegetable, diet are important too.

TREATMENT

+ **Poor memory and low concentration (for example, when studying and for exams)** Take ginkgo or *rhodiola* as concentrated extracts. Eat a sprig of fresh rosemary leaves or take 30 drops of rosemary tincture one to three times a day. These remedies can be combined.
+ **Poor memory linked to stress and anxiety** Take a lemon balm infusion. Make it using 10 g (⅓ oz) dried herb to 200 ml (7 fl oz) water. Take 2.5 ml (½ tsp) of lemon balm tincture three times a day. Take *rhodiola* as a concentrated extract. Eat a sprig of fresh rosemary leaves or take 30 drops of rosemary tincture one to three times a day. Take 20 drops of sage tincture one to three times a day.
+ **To support effective circulation within the brain** Consume up to 3 g (½ tsp) of cinnamon powder a day with food. Take ginkgo as a concentrated extract. Eat a sprig of fresh rosemary leaves or take 30 drops of rosemary tincture one to three times a day. Take *bilberry*, *grapeseed*, or *green tea* as concentrated extracts.
+ **For long-term treatment to protect against dementia** Take ginkgo as a concentrated extract. Take 2.5 ml (½ tsp) lemon balm tincture one to three times a day. Eat a sprig of fresh rosemary leaves or take 30 drops of rosemary tincture one to three times a day. Take *bilberry*, *grapeseed*, or *green tea* as concentrated extracts and 10 saffron strands a day.

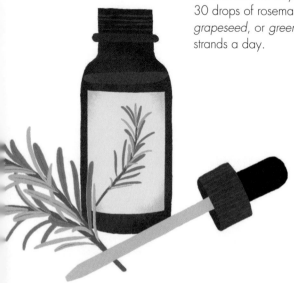

SHINGLES

The herpes zoster virus that causes chickenpox also causes this disease. You should start treatment as soon as possible (whether with prescribed or herbal medicine). Treatment is likely to be most effective when the affected nerve tissue, immune resistance, and nutritional status are all supported. No single external remedy is guaranteed to work.

TREATMENT

+ Apply freshly squeezed ginger juice directly to sores. You can extract the juice by placing a piece of fresh ginger root in a garlic crusher.
+ Apply lemon balm cream or juice squeezed from a fresh leaf directly to sores.
+ Apply aloe vera gel or juice directly to sores.
+ Apply *neem* cream – use one that includes essential oils such as *ylang ylang* (neat *neem* oil has a very unpleasant odour).
+ Apply St John's wort as an infused oil or cream directly to sores.
+ Apply 1 drop of *geranium*, lavender, peppermint, or thyme essential oil to each sore or blend 10–15 drops per 10 ml (2 tsp) St John's wort infused oil.

The above remedies will also prove helpful for any pain that continues after the sores have healed (see also, Understanding Pain, p. 40).

INTERNAL TREATMENT

+ **For a tonic neuroprotective activity** Take a lemon balm, rosemary, or thyme infusion. Make it using 5–10 g (2½–5 tsp) dried herb to 200 ml (7 fl oz) water. Or take 5 ml (1 tsp) of lemon balm, rosemary, and thyme tincture, in equal parts, three times a day.
+ **To support nerve resistance** Take St John's wort as a concentrated extract or take 30 drops of tincture three times a day.
+ **While the infection is present** Take 2.5 ml (½ tsp) echinacea and/or olive leaf tincture two to three times a day.
+ **To control inflammation** Take 2–4 g (½–1 tsp) of turmeric powder or take *boswellia* or turmeric as concentrated extracts.
+ **To improve vitality and immune function** Take adaptogens maca, ashwagandha, *gotu kola*, Korean ginseng, and/or *rhodiola* – see Nervous Exhaustion and Tiredness for dosages, p. 89.

FROM THE GARDEN

+ Echinacea, lemon balm, rosemary, thyme

NERVE PAIN

Herbal remedies offer a valuable option when considering treatment for nerve pain, including post herpetic neuralgia and sciatica. The most powerful analgesics, such as morphine, are extracted from plants but the sedation and side-effects they cause counter-balance their effectiveness. The analgesic and anti-inflammatory remedies listed below are non-addictive and only cause drowsiness if taken to excess. This, however, means that you cannot expect them to provide the same degree of pain relief. Topical treatments applied to the skin can be very helpful and are often undervalued.

EXTERNAL TREATMENT

Apply the following remedies both to the site of pain and on affected nerve tissue. In sciatica, for example, which results from nerve compression in the lower back, apply to the lower back and down the back of the leg.

+ Healing Oil (see p. 83).
+ St John's wort cream or infused oil. Add in 5 drops of *clove*, *geranium*, or lavender essential oil per 10 ml (2 tsp) of cream or oil.
+ *Chilli* and ginger oil (see Infused Oils p. 236) or capsaicin cream (extracted from chillies). Both sting intensely to begin with but then block pain perception; the latter is more effective and your doctor can prescribe it for you.
+ *Neem* cream and oil and CBD (*cannabidiol*) cream or oil may help in both acute and chronic nerve pain.

INTERNAL TREATMENT

+ **To support nerve repair** Take 30 drops of St John's wort tincture three times a day, or take St John's wort as a concentrated extract.
+ **To relax spinal muscles and reduce inflammation and nerve compression in the case of sciatica** Take 2.5 ml (½ tsp) of cramp bark tincture one to five times a day.
+ **To ease nerve pain** Take anti-inflammatory *boswellia*, turmeric, or *willow bark* as concentrated extracts.
+ Take 5 ml (1 tsp) of lavender, passion flower, or valerian tincture up to three times a day (tinctures can be single or combined), or take as concentrated extracts. All have analgesic activity.
+ Take *cannabidiol* (CBD) oil extracts.
+ Adaptogens ashwagandha, *gotu kola*, maca, Korean ginseng, and/or *rhodiola* can also help – see Nervous Exhaustion and Tiredness for dosages, p. 89.

Circulatory System

When thinking about the cardiovascular system, the focus tends to be on the heart and the arteries – the dynamic, high-pressure parts of the system that are essential to life. When things go wrong here, life-threatening problems such as heart attack and stroke can result. Yet true cardiovascular health depends just as much on the capillaries, the network of micro-tubules that carries blood and oxygen to tissues throughout the body and that, if put end to end, would measure roughly 50,000 km (31,000 miles) in length.

Poor blood flow and poor function in this vast network may not directly cause life-threatening illness, but they do contribute to many chronic health problems, especially chronic inflammatory conditions, such as type 2 diabetes. This remarkable network of capillaries ensures that tissues throughout the body have access to oxygen, glucose, and nutrients – and that waste products can be efficiently removed. Many herbs and foods contain compounds, notably flavonoids, that support capillary health. Attending to the health of the circulatory system as a whole may be the single most important physical factor in ageing well and in preventing the onset of both acute problems such as heart attack and chronic problems such dementia. The suggestions that follow in this section are for non-life-threatening circulatory problems. A herbal practitioner or naturopath may well be able to provide safe and effective treatment in more serious conditions.

COLD PERIPHERIES AND CHILBLAINS

Poor circulation to the hands and feet (and nose and head) is a common problem. Understood by herbalists as a cold, deficient condition, herbs that promote effective peripheral circulation are mostly warming or hot in character, adding "fire" to the circulation and opening up peripheral blood vessels, so that blood is more able to reach the peripheries.

EXTERNAL TREATMENT

+ Rub fresh ginger juice into chilblains. You can extract the juice by placing a chunk of fresh root in a garlic crusher.
+ Apply 1 drop of propolis tincture or (better) a propolis cream/balm to the site.
+ Peppermint oil can relieve pain.

INTERNAL TREATMENT

+ Consume hot spices routinely through the winter months. Add fresh and dried ginger root and *chilli* powder or sauce to meals. Take 2–4 g (½–1 tsp) of cinnamon powder a day.
+ **To strengthen peripheral circulation** Take ginkgo as a concentrated extract. Or take 2.5 g (½ tsp) of hawthorn leaf or berry powder or 2.5 ml (½ tsp) of hawthorn tincture once or twice a day. Or take 20–30 drops of angelica root tincture two to three times a day.
+ **To improve general circulation** Take a *lime flower* infusion and 30 drops of *yarrow* tincture twice a day. Make the infusion using 5–10 g (2½–5 tsp) dried herb to 200 ml (7 fl oz) water. You can take both long-term.
+ Take *bilberry*, *grapeseed*, or *green tea* as concentrated extracts.
+ If low blood pressure is also a problem, see p. 96.

FROM THE GARDEN

+ Hawthorn

HIGH BLOOD PRESSURE

A natural approach to treating high blood pressure involves combining lifestyle changes, such as including eating a Mediterranean-type diet along with appropriate herbal medicines and supplements. Each element in such a regime contributes a small percentage effect towards the objective of normalizing blood pressure. For example, garlic taken long-term at the right dosage will help to lower blood pressure by about 10 per cent. Other remedies, such as hawthorn and olive leaf, can produce similar results. Taken together with lifestyle changes, such as breathing exercises that ease internal pressure, there is a cumulative effect that leads to improved efficiency in heart and circulatory function.

+ Include raw and cooked *beetroot, carrot, celery,* fennel, garlic, and *onions* regularly in the diet. Make a smoothie. Drink a glass of *beetroot* juice daily. Include olive oil in your diet. Restrict salt intake. Avoid alcohol.
+ **To lower raised blood pressure** Take a *lime flower* and/or *hibiscus* flower infusion. Make it using 10 g (⅓ oz) dried herb to 200 ml (7 fl oz) water. Both are pleasant to drink.
+ **For high blood pressure** Take 2.5 ml (½ tsp) of hawthorn, fennel seed, olive leaf, and/or cramp bark tincture once or twice a day. These are key herbs. For a good combination, take 5 ml (1 tsp) of hawthorn, fennel seed, and cramp bark tincture in equal parts, two to three times a day.
+ Take *bilberry, grapeseed,* or *green tea* as concentrated extracts and consume red and purple fruits and vegetables.

FROM THE GARDEN   + Hawthorn, lemon balm

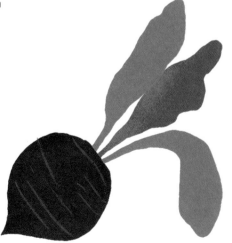

LOW BLOOD PRESSURE

Though it may seem contrary, hawthorn – one of the best remedies for high blood pressure – is also a key herb for low blood pressure. Research indicates that hawthorn berry and leaf support the heart and circulation in functioning with greater efficiency, whether this involves relaxing an over-pressurized system (as in high blood pressure) or toning up an underactive system. Several other herbs also work to promote more efficient blood flow around the body, helping to underpin stamina and vitality.

+ Take 2.5 g (½ tsp) of hawthorn powder once or twice a day or 2.5 ml (½ tsp) of hawthorn tincture two to three times a day.
+ Eat a sprig of fresh rosemary leaves, or take 30 drops of rosemary tincture once or twice a day.
+ Take a nettle infusion. Make it using 10 g (⅓ oz) dried herb to 200 ml (7 fl oz) water. Take 2.5 ml (½ tsp) of nettle tincture two to three times a day.
+ Enrich your diet with fresh and dried ginger root.

FROM THE GARDEN   + Hawthorn, nettle, rosemary

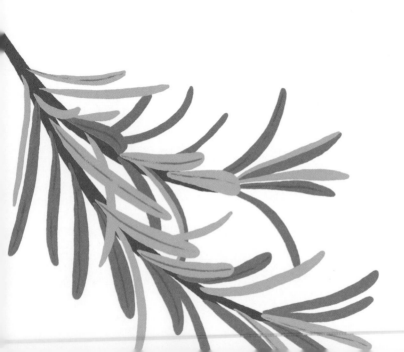

PALPITATIONS

Palpitations can be very disturbing but are usually a mild, short-term problem. Where palpitations are severe, last more than five minutes, or recur frequently, seek professional advice. The following remedies can be very helpful in relieving this problem.

TREATMENT	+ Massage a few drops of neat lavender or peppermint essential oil into the back of the neck and temples.
	+ **To stabilize the heartbeat and relieve associated anxiety** Take 20–30 drops of *lime flower*, lemon balm, or passion flower tincture in water every hour (singly or as a combination of two or more). It is best to sip this and retain it in the mouth to encourage oral absorption. Limit treatment to a maximum of ten doses a day.
	+ **To improve heart regularity and reduce irritability** Take ginkgo as a concentrated extract or take 2.5 ml (½ tsp) of hawthorn and olive leaf tincture in equal parts, one to three times a day. These are best taken at a low dosage long-term.
FROM THE GARDEN	+ Hawthorn, lemon balm

VARICOSE VEINS, THREAD VEINS, AND HAEMORRHOIDS

Venous problems are often allowed to deteriorate until a point where surgery becomes necessary. If started early enough, herbal medicine can be extremely useful in stabilizing, and sometimes healing, venous problems, though remedies generally need to be taken long-term to achieve good results. Treatments typically used for venous problems can also prove helpful in relieving restless legs.

TREATMENT

+ **To soothe, tighten, and stimulate repair of varicose veins, haemorrhoids, and thread veins** Apply aloe vera, horse chestnut, or witch hazel lotion or cream morning and evening.
+ Take horse chestnut – the key remedy for venous problems – and ginkgo as concentrated extracts, plus *bilberry*, *grapeseed*, or *green tea* as concentrated extracts. This combination can also help with restless legs.

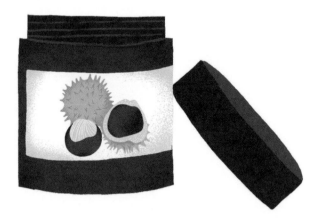

NOSEBLEEDS

Several herbs will help to stop a nosebleed, along with the traditional cold compress on the back of the neck. If a nosebleed continues unchecked despite treatment, or if nosebleeds recur, seek professional advice. Note also that nosebleeds are far more likely to occur if you are taking anticoagulants.

TREATMENT

+ Soak a small piece of cotton wool in witch hazel water and use this to plug the affected nostril(s).
+ Take a *yarrow* infusion. Make it using 5 g (2½ tsp) dried herb to 200 ml (7 fl oz) water and brew it for 15 minutes. Take 30 drops of *yarrow* tincture every 30 minutes (up to six doses in a day).
+ Take a nettle infusion. Make it using 10 g (⅓ oz) dried herb to 200 ml (7 fl oz) water and brew it for 15 minutes. Take 5 ml (1 tsp) of nettle tincture every 30 minutes (up to six doses in a day).

EASY BRUISING

Easy bruising may be a sign of capillary fragility, the result of vitamin B12 or K deficiency, of medication that thins the blood (including herbs, such as garlic and ginkgo), or of a blood disorder. Seek professional advice for large or repeated bruising that cannot be explained by accidental injury. For the best results, you will usually need to continue treatment long-term

TREATMENT

+ Apply arnica lotion or cream, comfrey ointment or cream, or horse chestnut lotion or cream to the affected area. See also, Bruises and Sprains, p. 70.
+ Take 2.5 ml (½ tsp) of *yarrow* and nettle tincture in equal parts twice a day.
+ Take *bilberry*, *grapeseed*, or *green tea* as concentrated extracts.

Respiratory System

Though we do not generally think about it, the respiratory system that draws air in from the nose and warms and moistens it on the way down into the lobes of the lungs is an interface between the outside world and our own internal environment. It is designed to fulfil two competing objectives – to maximize the exchange of gases, and to minimize the risk of infection from airborne particles. Key to this task are the mucous membranes – an internal "skin" that lines the entire respiratory tract. For effective respiratory function, it is essential that mucous membranes are healthy. Like skin, they prevent bacteria and other infectious agents entering the bloodstream but they also trap dust, air pollution, and pathogens in their sticky mucus lining. When mucous membranes become too dry or congested, they cease to be able to function properly and allergy, infection, and chronic catarrhal states are likely to develop.

SNEEZING, HAY FEVER, AND ALLERGIC SYMPTOMS

Allergic symptoms such as sneezing, running nose and eyes, and chronic congestion indicate mucous membranes that are struggling to maintain normal function. Removing yourself as far as possible from allergens makes obvious sense, but avoiding sugar and alcohol and keeping the nasal and sinus passages moist are important as well. The following herbs moisten and tighten or tone up lax mucous membranes, strengthening their resistance to allergens and pathogens. For the best results take remedies consistently for several weeks.

TREATMENT	
	+ Take an elderflower and/or plantain infusion. Make it using 10 g (⅓ oz) dried herb to 200 ml (7 fl oz) water. Add in 20–30 drops of liquorice tincture (up to three times a day). Chamomile and nettle infusions are also helpful.

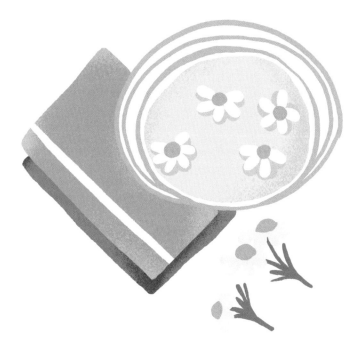

+ **Acute sneezing and rhinitis** Make a chamomile steam inhalation by infusing 10 g (⅓ oz) dried flowers in 200 ml (7 fl oz) water. Place the infusion in a bowl, cover your head with a cloth, and inhale the steam for five minutes.
+ **Nasal and sinus irritation** Suck up *beetroot* juice through a wide straw into the nasal passages. This is slightly unusual but nonetheless comforting! You can also use salt water, but this can be too drying.
+ **In difficult cases** Take 2.5 ml (½ tsp) of nettle and echinacea tincture in equal parts, two to four times a day.

UPPER RESPIRATORY INFECTION

Many herbs help to prevent upper respiratory infections, and to speed recovery should an infection occur. A herbal approach focuses on supporting respiratory mucous membrane resistance and body-wide immune function. Chronic weakness in mucous membrane function makes it easier for pathogens to enter the bloodstream, meaning that an infection can more readily become systemic. Enhancing systemic immune function helps to block viral entry into cells and slow viral and bacterial replication. See also, Colds and Flu and Covid-19, pp. 103 and 104.

GENERAL REMEDIES

+ Take an elderflower (two parts), peppermint (two parts), and *yarrow* (one part) infusion. Make it using 15–20 g (½–¾ oz) dried herb to 400 ml (14 fl oz) water. Drink it hot, in divided doses. This traditional combination ("cold flu tea") is a favourite for cold and flu symptoms and will speed recovery. It is especially useful in fever, as all three herbs cool the body and stimulate sweating. To strengthen sweating and bring down a fever, add a pinch of *chilli* powder or a few drops of *chilli* tincture/sauce to the infusion. Sweeten with honey. This infusion can also be inhaled.
+ Propolis is exceptionally useful for upper respiratory infections. A potent antiseptic and antioxidant, propolis tightens up mucous membranes and their ability to resist viral and bacterial infection. Use it sparingly – 5–10 drops in an infusion is a good way to take it. For sore throats, buy propolis in a spray bottle. As Covid-19 infection mostly depends on viral entry through mucous membranes in the nose and throat, propolis may help to prevent Covid infection. It is certainly useful in treating colds, flu, and Covid-19 symptoms.
+ Herbal anti-inflammatories such as *boswellia*, turmeric, and *willow bark* help to control inflammation and relieve symptoms caused by infection. You can take each of them as a concentrated extract, much as you might take a paracetamol to control fever and ease pain. All three may help to prevent inflammatory damage in Covid infection.
+ Infused *chilli* and ginger oil (see Hot-Infused Oils, p. 236), and "hot" oils such as *tiger balm*, make excellent warming salves. Apply them to the skin for sinus aches and chesty conditions, but use them sparingly.
+ **For chest infections** Make an *onion* poultice: chop two *onions* and simmer gently in a saucepan with a little water for two to three minutes. Pour the contents of the saucepan into a clean dishcloth and fold to make a square poultice. Hold this on the chest for 20 minutes.

COLDS AND FLU

All of the remedies listed on pp. 102 will prove useful in aiding recovery. It is good to explore what works for you – use the remedies that you find work well or feel best about using.

ADDITIONAL MEASURES	+ **To help control fever and reduce recovery time** Take elderberry as a concentrated extract (good for children in liquid forms). Take a stronger-acting *yarrow* infusion. Make it using 5–7.5 g (2½–3 tsp) dried herb to 200 ml (7 fl oz) water and add a pinch of *chilli* powder to stimulate increased sweating, as wanted.
	+ Take echinacea as a concentrated extract or take 2.5 ml (½ tsp) of echinacea tincture two to four times a day for up to seven days. Echinacea is best taken in combination with other remedies, for example, with an elderflower infusion or elderberry extract.
	+ *African geranium* (*Pelargonium sidoides*) extract is a safe and useful remedy for colds and flu in adults and children.
FROM THE GARDEN	+ Echinacea, elderflower or berry
THE KITCHEN BREW	+ Simple ingredients from the kitchen can make very useful medicines to treat colds, sore throats, and flu-like symptoms.
	+ Place the following in a mug: a large garlic clove (chopped or crushed), a fingertip-sized piece of fresh ginger root (chopped or grated), fresh *lemon* or *lime* juice, 5 ml (1 tsp) of honey. Pour on water just off the boil. Stir, leave for a minute or two, and sip the remedy, if possible eating the contents at the bottom.
	+ Optional additional spices: 2.5 g (½ tsp) of *black pepper*; a pinch of *chilli*; 2.5 g (½ tsp) of cinnamon; 5 *cloves*; 5 g (1 tsp) of fresh or dried turmeric root.

COVID-19

Natural remedies such as propolis may possibly reduce the risk of developing a Covid-19 infection, but more realistically, herbal remedies are likely to reduce symptom severity and shorten the time taken to recover. All remedies listed on pp. 102–103 will provide some benefit in Covid infection, strengthening immune resistance, countering infection, and easing symptoms. From preliminary research, the following herbs appear to have direct activity against Covid infection, helping to block the virus' ability to "dock" on specific cell receptor sites.

TREATMENT	+ Take a *yarrow* infusion. Make it using 5–7.5 g (2½–3 tsp) dried herb to 200 ml (7 fl oz) water. + Take a *hibiscus* infusion. Make it using 10 g (⅓ oz) dried herb to 200 ml (7 fl oz) water. + Take 2 g (½ tsp) of ground milk thistle seed a day or take milk thistle as a concentrated extract. + Take 20 drops of barberry tincture two to four times a day (this has a very bitter taste). + Take 10 drops of liquorice tincture one to three times a day.
ADDITIONAL MEASURES	+ Take 2–4 g (½–1 tsp) of turmeric powder a day or take turmeric as a concentrated extract. + Consume fruit/freshly squeezed citrus juice. + Consume a crushed garlic clove a day or take garlic as a concentrated extract. + **Where the chest and breathing are affected** Self-help measures include massaging *chilli-* and ginger-infused oil, *tiger balm*, or Healing Oil (see p. 83) into the chest. Or apply a warm *onion* poultice (see p. 102). Make sure to keep warm.

SINUS PROBLEMS AND CATARRH

Low-level infection, environmental pollutants, dehydration, food sensitivity, and allergy can all cause nasal congestion, sinus headache, and lowered immune resistance. Steam inhalation can bring temporary relief. Long-term treatment aims to restore effective immune function and healthy mucus secretions that are neither too watery nor too sticky.

TREATMENT	+ Take a chamomile and/or *eucalyptus* infusion or use it as a steam inhalation. Make it using 10 g (⅓ oz) dried herb to 200 ml (7 fl oz) water. For a steam inhalation, pour the infusion into a bowl, cover your head with a cloth, and inhale the steam for five minutes. + Take 5 ml (1 tsp) of marigold, echinacea, and thyme tincture, in equal parts, five times a day (high dose for up to a week). This is a good combination to take in tandem with garlic and propolis. + **To relieve congestion and heal damaged mucous membranes** Take a *ground ivy* and/or plantain infusion. Make it using 10 g (⅓ oz) dried herb to 200 ml (7 fl oz) water. + Where mucous membranes are very dry, chia seeds and flaxseeds are useful. See Acid Indigestion, p. 115.
FROM THE GARDEN	+ Chamomile, *eucalyptus*, plantain, thyme

SORE THROAT AND HOARSENESS

Viral infections cause most sore throats. Combining local treatment, in particular gargling, with general immune support is likely to be most effective, though gargling (or a throat spray) can be sufficient. Gargle away for two to three minutes before swallowing a remedy.

TREATMENT	+ Make a sage infusion using 5 g (2½ tsp) dried or 10 g (⅓ oz) fresh herb to 200 ml (7 fl oz) water and steeping for 10 minutes. Use warm as a gargle. To increase its strength, add a few drops of *chilli* sauce. Alternative herbs include *blackberry leaf*, *raspberry leaf*, and thyme. + **Hoarseness and loss of voice** Take a plantain infusion. Make it using 10 g (⅓ oz) dried herb to 200 ml (7 fl oz) water. A propolis spray is convenient, particularly when out of the house. + **Dry mucous membranes** Chia seeds and flaxseeds are useful. See Acid Indigestion, p. 115.

TONSILLITIS

Tonsillitis is a bacterial infection of the tonsils that needs immediate effective treatment. If you do not feel confident in treating it, seek professional advice. Gargles will be helpful (see Sore Throat and Hoarseness, p. 105).

TREATMENT	+ Take echinacea as a concentrated extract or take 5 ml (1 tsp) of echinacea tincture once or twice a day for up to seven days. + Take elderberry as a concentrated extract up to five times a day. Gargle it with 10 drops of propolis in warm water, then swallow. + Take 5 ml (1 tsp) of thyme (two parts), rosemary (two parts), barberry (2 parts), and liquorice (one part) tincture three to five times a day, for up to seven days at higher dose. Dilute the combined tincture in warm water, gargle, then swallow. + Regularly take garlic as crushed cloves or as a concentrated extract.
FROM THE GARDEN	+ Echinacea, plantain, rosemary, sage, thyme

PAINFUL DRY COUGHS

A cough is the body's attempt to clear an irritant or mucus from the airways. A cough can be dry and irritable – coming from the throat and trachea – or, as in bronchitis, moist and "productive", with plenty of phlegm (see p. 109). Demulcent, moistening herbs, such as flaxseeds and chia seeds, are best used for dry, irritable coughs.

TREATMENT	+ Place 2 g (½ tsp) of *marshmallow* leaf/powdered root, flaxseeds, or chia seeds in a glass of warm water. Stir well and leave for 30 minutes. The water will become gooey (the chia seeds will look like frogspawn). Add honey and drink slowly. This can be very helpful in easing painful coughs. + Take a *ground ivy* and/or plantain infusion. Make it using 10 g (⅓ oz) dried herb to 200 ml (7 fl oz) water. + Take 2.5 ml (½ tsp) of thyme (three parts) and liquorice (one part) tincture up to four times a day.
FROM THE GARDEN	+ Plantain, thyme

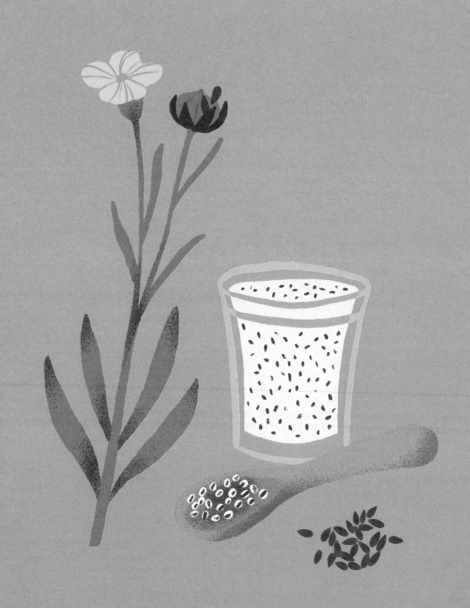

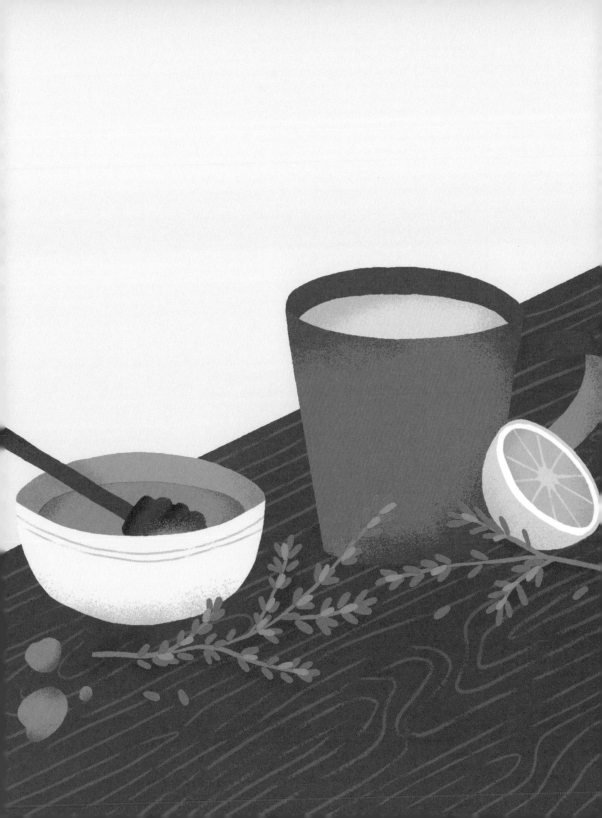

PRODUCTIVE COUGH AND BRONCHITIS

Mucusy coughs and those associated with bronchitis generally need expectorants, such as elecampane, to stimulate clearance of mucus from the chest.

TREATMENT

+ Make a *eucalyptus* and/or thyme infusion using 10 g (⅓ oz) dried herb to 200 ml (7 fl oz) water. Inhale the steam before drinking.
+ Massage *chilli-* and ginger-infused oil, *tiger balm*, or Healing Oil (see p. 83) into the chest, especially before going to bed.
+ **Bronchitis and sensitivity to the cold** Take 5 ml (1 tsp) of angelica root, echinacea, and elecampane tincture, in equal parts, with warm water, one to three times a day.

FROM THE GARDEN

+ Echinacea, *eucalyptus*, thyme

ASTHMA

Asthma can be a severely troubling condition and generally requires professional advice and treatment. With asthma, the aim is always to maintain a symptom-free state rather than to have occasional bouts that need urgent treatment. In mild cases, herbal remedies may be sufficient to remain symptom free, but the herbs listed here can all be safely combined with prescribed asthma medication, where necessary, including inhalers.

+ Take a thyme infusion. Make it using 5 g (2½ tsp) dried herb to 200 ml (7 fl oz) water and honey.
+ Take an elderflower or *white horehound* infusion. Make it using 10 g (⅓ oz) dried herb to 200 ml (7 fl oz) water and honey.
+ Take 2.5 ml (½ tsp) of angelica root (one part) and cramp bark (two parts) tincture up to six times a day for up to one week. If you do not have angelica root, just use cramp bark.
+ **To ease discomfort and distress** Take 20 drops of valerian tincture, as wanted, with water.

+ Elderflower, thyme

Digestion and Gut Health

Our digestive system is home to around 400 different species of bacteria, with a total population of more than 30 trillion cells making up the gut flora or microbiome, and has the capacity to process almost anything we swallow – food and drink, contaminants, and infectious organisms. Roughly 9 m (30 ft) in length, the digestive tract extracts goodness from our diets and regularly removes waste products and dead bacteria in our stools. This is done with such efficiency that, most of the time, we are unaware of it working away to ensure that we have the necessary nutrition to maintain life, health, and well-being.

The digestive tract is really a hollow tube that runs from the mouth to the anus. Lined with mucous membranes that act as an "internal skin", it has its own nervous system (the gut brain), along with specialized areas such as the stomach and small intestine that secrete essential digestive juices. The gut brain controls the rate and pace of movement of food through the gut, and selectively controls digestion and absorption of nutrients across the gut wall into the bloodstream. The contents of the gut are policed by a vast immune system to prevent infection and inflammation – 75 per cent of the body's immune cells are located in the digestive tract.

We notice absence more than presence – in this case, we only take note of our digestion when it is no longer functioning effectively and we experience unwanted symptoms. Most digestive symptoms, such as nausea, acid indigestion, and constipation, are functional and result from emotional or physical interference in the gut's regular pattern of activity. The gut needs the body and mind to be relaxed to process foods efficiently. When we are stressed, blood flows to the muscles and away from the digestive tract, reducing the level of digestive secretions. Eating regular meals in a relaxed environment allows healthy digestion to take place and can reverse problems with digestive function. Herbs can be highly effective in restoring normal gut activity – remedies such as chamomile, fennel, and peppermint stimulate digestive secretions and soothe inflammation and nerve endings in the gut wall. Marigold, meadowsweet, and plantain promote tissue healing and counter inflammation.

A healthy gut flora, or microbiome, is also a key factor in digestive health. A harmful mix of gut bacteria is associated with many chronic inflammatory problems, including irritable bowel syndrome and ulcerative colitis, as well as type 2 diabetes, depression, and allergies such as eczema. Improving digestive function and elimination stimulates a healthier, more balanced gut flora. Some herbs such as garlic, ginger, and turmeric are notable for their ability to support a healthy gut flora.

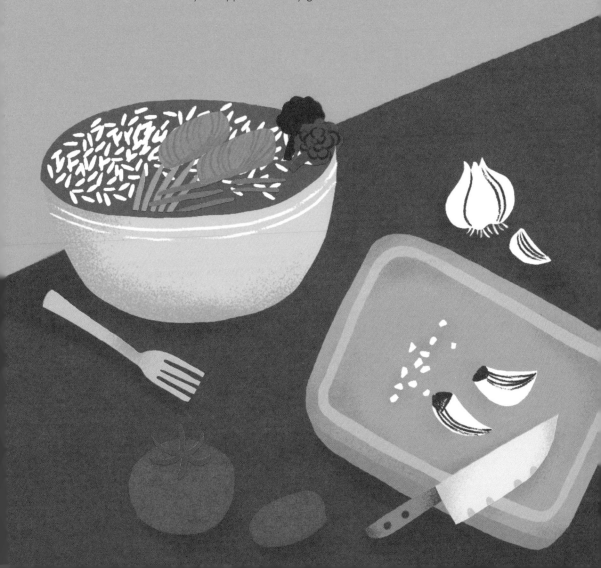

HICCUPS

Hiccups result from irritation of the vagus nerve and usually clear of their own accord. There are many home remedies for hiccups, but no one treatment is uniquely effective.

TREATMENT

+ Sip a cold chamomile, cramp bark, or peppermint infusion. Make it using 5–10 g (2½–5 tsp) dried herb to 200 ml (7 fl oz) water. Take 2.5 ml (½ tsp) of chamomile, cramp bark, or peppermint tincture up to six times a day or sip diluted in water.
+ Where hiccups recur repeatedly, take a regular peppermint infusion or take 2.5 ml (½ tsp) of cramp bark tincture twice a day.
+ A few drops of lavender or peppermint essential oil rubbed on the back of the neck can prove helpful.

FROM THE GARDEN

+ Chamomile, lavender, peppermint

STOMACH ACHE

Many herbs can help soothe stomach ache and settle the digestion, relieving a sense of fullness or discomfort. Herbs suggested here will warm and relax the stomach and counter inflammation. Stomach ache may occur as a symptom in many conditions – see also, Acid Indigestion, p. 115, Gastrointestinal Infection, p. 114, and Weak Digestion, p. 117.

TREATMENT

+ **For symptomatic relief** Take a cinnamon, ginger, and turmeric infusion. Use grated fresh root, a teabag, or 2 g (½ tsp) of powder for each herb and infuse in 200 ml (7 fl oz) water for five to 10 minutes. Squeeze in fresh lemon juice and sweeten with honey, as wanted.
+ **To soothe mild indigestion and stomach ache** Take a chamomile and/or meadowsweet infusion. Make it using 2–3 teabags brewed in a cup or 10 g (⅓ oz) dried herb to 200 ml (7 fl oz) water. Or take 20 drops of liquorice tincture one to three times a day.

NAUSEA AND VOMITING

Many different factors, including anxiety, infection, and motion sickness, can produce the classic sense of digestive dis-ease that is the mark of nausea. Nerve irritation, typically of the vagus nerve, causes nausea, which has symptoms that include dizziness, tinnitus, and sweating. A combination of chamomile and ginger can bring prompt relief to these unpleasant symptoms and may ease the sense of needing to vomit.

TREATMENT	+ Make a warm infusion of chamomile and ginger by steeping 10 g (⅓ oz) dried flowers and a 2 cm (¾ in) piece ginger root (chopped) in 200 ml (7 fl oz) water for 10 minutes. Add lemon juice and sweeten with honey, and sip it. Other herbs to use include *cardamom*, cinnamon, peppermint, and turmeric.
	+ Make a warm infusion of *marshmallow* root powder mixed into a liquid paste with warm water. Take small amounts as wanted.
	+ To help relieve nausea, massage a few drops of lavender or peppermint essential oil into the back of the neck.
FROM THE GARDEN	+ Chamomile, *marshmallow*, lavender, peppermint

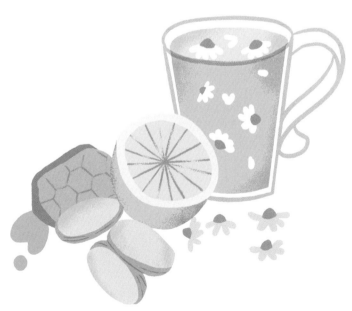

GASTROINTESTINAL INFECTION AND FOOD POISONING

Herbs and spices generally provide effective treatment for digestive infections and can help keep fever, pain, cramps, and diarrhoea under control. If you are suffering from high fever and have acute, uncontrolled diarrhoea, seek professional treatment.

Cooking with plenty of herbs and spices, such as *cardamom*, *cloves*, and ginger, is a good way to reduce your chances of developing food poisoning and these remedies are equally important in treating instances of gastrointestinal infection. Infusions with added honey and *lemon* or *lime* juice help to recoup fluid lost through diarrhoea.

TREATMENT	+ Garlic is the key herb for digestive infection. Infuse 2–3 crushed garlic cloves in 200 ml (7 fl oz) water, along with 5 g (1 tsp) cinnamon and/or 4–5 *cloves*. Sip warm, sweetened with honey.
	+ **To help control inflammation and diarrhoea** Take up to 15 ml (1 tbsp) of aloe vera juice three times a day. Take a sage infusion. Make it using 5 g (2½ tsp) herb in 200 ml (7 fl oz) water.
	+ **For additional antibacterial and antiviral support** Take 2.5ml (½ tsp) of barberry, marigold, echinacea, or olive leaf tincture (twice a day for a single herb and up to four times a day for combined herbs).
FROM THE GARDEN	+ Marigold, echinacea, garlic, sage

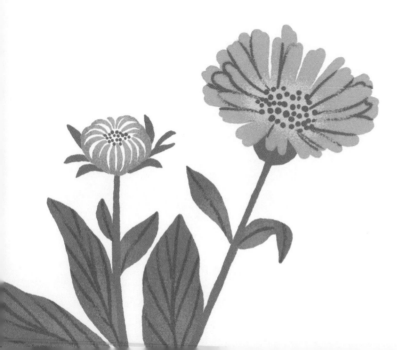

ACID INDIGESTION AND REFLUX

You can usually resolve minor episodes of acid indigestion and heartburn quickly. However, gastro-oesophageal reflux (GORD) and chronic acid indigestion need time to heal effectively. In good health, the protective mucus lining that holds the stomach's hydrochloric acid (pH 1.5–3.5) is renewed every three to four days. Mucus cells in the lower oesophagus serve a similar role. Poor diet, infection, and chronic stress slow the rate of repair and mucus secretion, making tissue more vulnerable to acid irritation and erosion. Poor posture and obesity also increase back pressure, pushing acid up into the oesophagus. The key to treating GORD is to protect and strengthen the mucous membranes of the oesophagus and stomach, while controlling excess acid production.

TREATMENT	A regular intake of the following demulcent herbs should provide relief to burning symptoms. + Take chia seeds, flaxseeds, or *slippery elm* as ground seeds or powder. Add 5–10 g (1–2 tsp) to a glass of water or chamomile infusion, stir, and leave for 20 to 30 minutes. Stir again, dilute if wanted, and drink. This is best taken after meals three times a day.
ADDITIONAL MEASURES	Take herbs to speed up tissue healing and counter inflammation. + Take 25 ml (1½ tbsp) of aloe vera juice a day. It is best taken in three divided doses. + Take 10–20 drops of liquorice tincture in water, two to three times a day after meals. + Make a marigold, chamomile, meadowsweet, or plantain infusion using 10 g (⅓ oz) dried herb to 200 ml (7 fl oz) water. Make a *yarrow* infusion using 5 g (2½ tsp) dried herb to 200 ml (7 fl oz) water. Take your choice of infusion as three divided doses. + Take 5 ml (1 tsp) of marigold, chamomile, meadowsweet, or plantain tincture, diluted, two to four times a day. Take 2.5 ml (½ tsp) of *yarrow* tincture, diluted, two to three times a day. Doses apply to single herbs and to combinations of them.
FROM THE GARDEN	+ Marigold, chamomile, plantain, *yarrow*

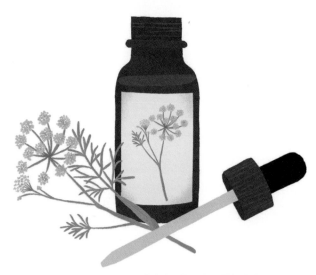

GAS, BLOATING, AND DISCOMFORT

Where these symptoms are occasional, causing minor discomfort, a simple approach is often sufficient. Eating slowly, chewing well, and adding more herbs and spices to your cooking or smoothies – for example, *caraway*, *cardamom*, or fennel seeds – can be enough to restore healthy digestive function. Ongoing bloating and discomfort requires a more intensive approach with tonics that stimulate the flow of digestive juices and support a healthy gut flora.

TREATMENT	+ **Occasional bloating** Take a chamomile infusion. Make it using 10 g (⅓ oz) dried herb to 200 ml (7 fl oz) water. Or take 2.5 ml (½ tsp) of chamomile tincture one to five times a day. Or take a fennel infusion. Make it using 5 g (2½ tsp) dried herb to 200 ml (7 fl oz) water. Or take 20 drops of fennel tincture one to four times a day. Add fresh ginger root to your diet. Take peppermint oil capsules (best taken 15 to 30 minutes before meals). + **Ongoing bloating and discomfort** Take 2.5 ml (½ tsp) of angelica, dandelion root, echinacea, or olive leaf tincture one to three times a day. Or take 1–2 crushed garlic cloves or take garlic as a concentrated extract. Take two or more of these herbs to counter harmful bacterial overgrowth, reduce gas levels, and gradually restore healthy digestive function.
FROM THE GARDEN	+ Chamomile, dandelion root, echinacea, fennel

WEAK DIGESTION AND POOR ABSORPTION

If you have a poor appetite, or despite eating well don't feel that this results in good energy levels, your digestive system might well need strengthening. Herbal remedies are unrivalled in this situation, improving blood flow to the gut, stimulating the flow of digestive juices, and enhancing nutrient absorption.

TREATMENT

+ Take one to three of the following herbs as tinctures two to three times a day (best 30 minutes before meals): 25 drops of angelica root, dandelion root, rosemary, or thyme tincture; 10–20 drops of liquorice tincture.
+ Include fresh or dried ginger root in your diet.

FROM THE GARDEN

+ Dandelion root, rosemary, thyme

CONSTIPATION

Whether a short- or long-term problem, adequate fluid intake is essential for constipation. Dehydration within the colon leads to a dry, hard-to-pass stool, which can act as a plug. Drink 1–2 litres (2–3½ pints) of water a day, and more in hot weather. Eat plenty of fruits and vegetables and take probiotics. Exercise is important, especially of the lower back and abdomen.

TREATMENT

+ For a gentle laxative, blend 2–3 fresh or dried *figs* and ½ tsp *tamarind* fruit or paste into a smoothie.
+ **To stimulate bowel contractions** Try *Chinese rhubarb* and *senna* – strong-acting herbs that can be effective 8 to 12 hours after ingestion. Take as concentrated extracts for a maximum of 10 days. *Senna* is best taken with ginger to reduce griping. You can buy *fig*, *tamarind*, and *Chinese rhubarb* as wrapped cubes (like stock cubes). These are excellent over-the-counter remedies for constipation.
+ **Chronic constipation** Chia seed, flaxseed, and *slippery elm* powder can be helpful. See Acid Indigestion, p. 115.
+ **Irritable bowel-type constipation with tensed colonic muscles due to inflammation and/or anxiety** Take aloe vera, chamomile, and cramp bark. See Diarrhoea, Looseness, and Urgency, p. 118, for dosages.

DIARRHOEA, LOOSENESS, AND URGENCY

An acute bout of diarrhoea is a sign that the body is trying to clear irritants or toxins from the gut. Supporting this cleansing process, while controlling looseness and urgency, is usually the best strategy. Chronic diarrhoea may be more complex to treat and a sign of irritable bowel syndrome or dysbiosis (poor gut bacterial balance). Dietary change and probiotics are often important here. Where infection is present, see Gastrointestinal Infection, p. 114. Herbal approaches aim to block nerve over-sensitivity within the gut, soothe gut wall irritability, and reduce the watery discharge of diarrhoea.

TREATMENT	+ Take a *clove* infusion. Make it using 2.5–5 g (1–2½ tsp) of *cloves* in 200 ml (7 fl oz) water and sip through the day. Or take 20 drops of *clove* tincture up to four times a day, or chew a whole *clove*. Or take a peppermint infusion. Make it using 10 g (⅓ oz) dried herb to 200 ml (7 fl oz) water. Or take peppermint essential oil capsules. Or take 2.5 ml (½ tsp) of peppermint tincture up to three times a day. + **To reduce fluid secretions** Take a meadowsweet and/or plantain infusion. Make it using 10 g (⅓ oz) dried herb to 200 ml (7 fl oz) water. Or take 2.5 ml (½ tsp) of meadowsweet and/or plantain tincture up to six times a day. Or take a sage infusion. Make it using 5 g (2½ tsp) dried herb to 200 ml (7 fl oz) water. Or take 20 drops of sage tincture up to five times a day. These are all astringent herbs. + Take 15 ml (1 tbsp) of aloe vera juice two to three times a day. Or take *boswellia* as a concentrated extract. Or take a chamomile infusion. Make it using 10 g (⅓ oz) dried herb to 200 ml (7 fl oz) water. Or take 2.5 ml (½ tsp) of chamomile tincture up five times a day. + Chia, flaxseed, and *slippery elm* powder can be extremely helpful. See Acid Indigestion, p. 115.
FROM THE GARDEN	+ Chamomile, peppermint, plantain, sage

Liver Function

The liver has many functions and, as its name suggests, good liver health is essential for vitality. It is unique among organs in that it is able to regrow, even after 90 per cent of it has been removed. Key liver activities include the storage of fat-soluble vitamins, the production of glycogen – a main store of energy within the body – and detoxification of hormones, waste products, and toxins. Herbalists look to the liver as an overall indicator of health and prescribe herbs specifically to promote liver function, which in turn supports health and vitality in other areas of the body.

In tandem with the pancreas, the liver is directly involved in maintaining stable blood glucose and blood cholesterol levels. As is well known, chronically raised or disordered blood glucose or blood cholesterol levels lead, over time, to the most common, serious health problems of our day – type 2 diabetes, atheroma, and raised blood pressure, obesity, and fatty liver disease. Collectively, these conditions are known as "metabolic syndrome", as they occur when the body's metabolic capacity has been overwhelmed. These problems typically need professional advice and treatment but, with appropriate diet and lifestyle changes, the herbs and recipes suggested here can lead to a radical improvement in metabolic health.

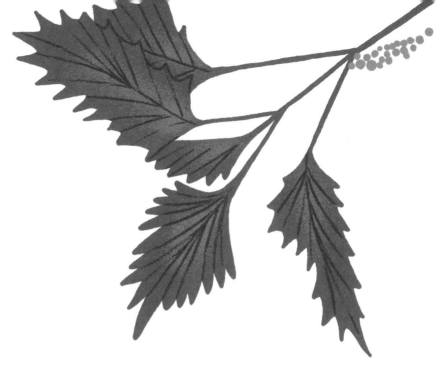

GLUCOSE METABOLISM

Many foods and herbs improve the ability of the pancreas and the liver to maintain healthy blood sugar levels. Some directly stimulate liver and pancreatic function, others slow absorption of sugars across the gut wall. It is best to take remedies at mealtimes. If you take them routinely, they will aid your body in regaining balanced insulin and glucose levels.

TREATMENT	+ Take two or three of the following a day: 2.5–5 g (½–1 tsp) of *bitter melon* powder; 2.5 g (½ tsp) of cinnamon powder; 5 g (1 tsp) of dandelion root powder; fresh ginger root; 2 g (½ tsp) of ground milk thistle seed or milk thistle as a concentrated extract; 5 g (1 tsp) of nettle powder. Take each remedy in divided doses, three times a day, before or with meals. The doses listed are for taking just one herb. If you take two or more, lower the dose of each. Including ground chia seeds or flaxseeds in a daily smoothie will also encourage more stable blood sugar levels. + Take 10–30 g (⅓–1 oz) of ground chia seeds or 10 g (⅓ oz) of ground flaxseeds a day.
FROM THE GARDEN	+ Dandelion root, nettle

CHOLESTEROL LEVELS

If you have raised cholesterol levels, or too little of the "good" HDL cholesterol, the simplest advice is to follow a Mediterranean-type diet: plenty of vegetables, fruits, and nuts, and some meat and fish. Research indicates that this diet is more effective for most people than taking statins. Stress levels are a frequently overlooked factor in raised cholesterol levels. Chronic stress increases blood fat levels. Doing what you can to reduce stress in your daily life and taking relaxant remedies, such as ashwagandha and valerian, can be helpful when combined with herbs that promote balanced blood fat levels.

TREATMENT	+ Take any of the following daily: artichoke as a concentrated extract; 5–10 g (1–2 tsp) of dandelion root powder; garlic as cloves or garlic as a concentrated extract; 2 g (½ tsp) of ground milk thistle seed or milk thistle as a concentrated extract; 2.5 ml (½ tsp) of olive leaf tincture one to three times a day; eat a sprig of fresh rosemary leaves or take 2.5 ml (½ tsp) rosemary tincture once or twice a day; 2–4 g (½–1 tsp) of turmeric powder or turmeric as a concentrated extract. A "mix and match" approach is best here. For example, increase garlic and turmeric in the diet, while also taking artichoke as a concentrated extract and olive leaf tincture. For other suitable relaxant herbs, see Irritability and Anger, p. 135.
	+ To slow the absorption of fats across the gut wall, take 10–30 g (⅓ –1 oz) of ground chia seeds or 10 g (⅓ oz) of ground flaxseeds a day.
FROM THE GARDEN	+ Dandelion root, garlic, rosemary

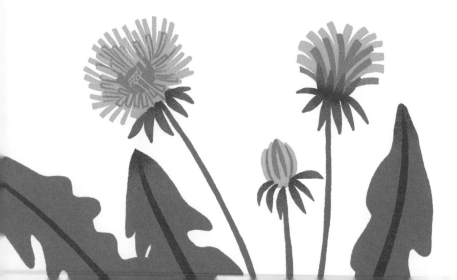

EXCESS WEIGHT

Losing excess weight is rarely easy and can be a dispiriting process. Navigating your way through the many different weight-loss regimes is also a challenge, with conflicting advice and raised expectations. A balanced approach to losing weight suggests that losing small amounts – 0.5–1 kg (1–2 lb) a week, month on month, works best. Liver and pancreatic health should improve with this approach and loss of muscle strength is unlikely to be a problem.

Whatever dietary regime you choose to follow, selected herbal remedies will work in tandem to aid weight loss by increasing metabolic rate, stimulating liver function, and working to stabilize blood glucose and cholesterol levels. Remedies such as rosemary and St John's wort can help by supporting a positive, focused mood.

TREATMENT

+ Recommended herbs include artichoke, *chilli*, cinnamon, dandelion, ginger, ginseng, milk thistle, olive leaf, rosemary, St John's wort, and turmeric. Read up about these herbs, note the recommended doses and select the ones that are the best fit for you, are affordable, and convenient to take. You will need to be comfortable about taking them long term.
+ If you only take one herb, fresh or dried rosemary might just be the best option.
+ Dandelion leaf is often recommended for weight loss, as its diuretic effect stimulates fluid loss. This is fine where fluid retention is a problem, but otherwise use dandelion root, which has a far more balanced effect in aiding weight loss.

FROM THE GARDEN

+ Dandelion, rosemary

EXCESS WEIGHT
PLAN

At least one liver herb (artichoke, dandelion, milk thistle, olive leaf, turmeric)   +   One hot, spicy herb (chilli sauce with meals or capsules, ginger, or rosemary)   +   One tonic herb (ginseng, rosemary, turmeric).

FATTY LIVER AND ABNORMAL LIVER FUNCTION

The liver is a sensitive organ. Only a few days of consuming a junk food diet will cause liver enzyme readings to rise, indicating that the liver is struggling. Over time, a high-fat, high-sugar, ultra-refined diet can result in major weight gain and fatty liver disease. Nevertheless, the good news is that the liver's remarkable capacity to regenerate means that there is always room to improve liver health, and herbal medicines are uniquely effective in this process.

TREATMENT

+ **To normalize liver function and support stable, balanced blood cholesterol and glucose levels** Take any of the following: artichoke as a concentrated extract; 5–10 g (1–2 tsp) of dandelion root powder or dandelion as a concentrated extract; 2 g (½ tsp) of ground milk thistle seed or milk thistle as a concentrated extract; olive leaf as a concentrated extract; 2–4 g (½–1 tsp) of turmeric powder or turmeric as a concentrated extract.
+ If you are going to take just one herb, go for artichoke. It is the best single remedy for fatty liver disease. Dandelion and milk thistle will help in all types of liver disease. Olive leaf and turmeric, like milk thistle, have potent antioxidant activity and support liver regeneration.

ADDITIONAL MEASURES

+ Take *bilberry*, *grapeseed*, or *green tea* as concentrated extracts. Consume 1–2 cloves garlic and/or 15 g (½ oz) of *goji berries* a day. Take 20 drops of liquorice tincture twice a day. These herbs add an extra dimension to the activity of the key liver herbs listed.

FROM THE GARDEN

+ Garlic, dandelion

A BALANCED TREATMENT PLAN

Take artichoke as a concentrated extract, ground milk thistle seeds, *bilberry* or *grapeseed* as concentrated extracts, and *goji berries*, while adding garlic and turmeric to food.

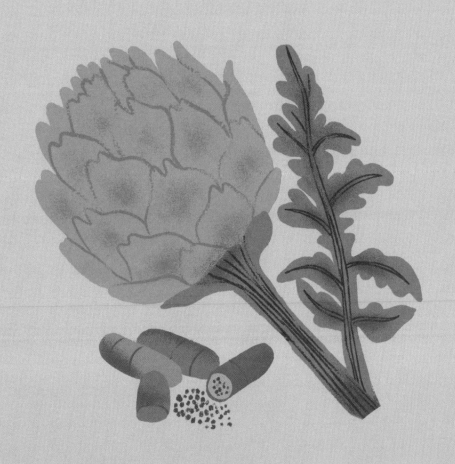

Urinary System

The kidneys are so effective in their role of filtering out water-soluble waste products that we remain unaware of their continuous work in cleansing and regulating fluid volumes within the body. The kidneys like water more than anything else and healthy renal and urinary tract function depends on a regular fluid intake. This intake should include 1–2 litres (1¾–3½ pints) water a day, which most of the time will maintain a healthy dilute urine. Dehydration (see also, Hydration p. 32) and a concentrated urine put the kidneys under stress and impair the urinary tract's capacity to resist inflammation and infection.

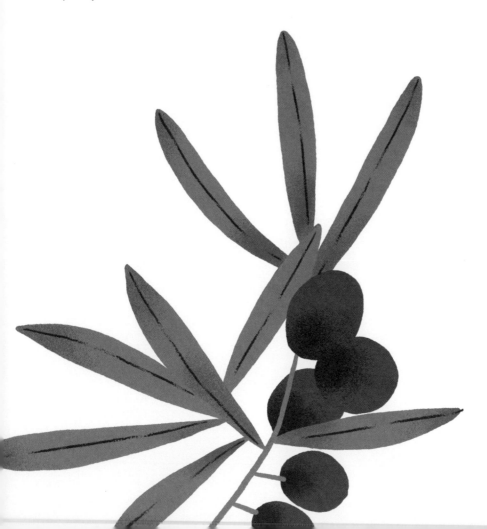

ACUTE CYSTITIS

Cystitis is a common bacterial infection that can be extremely unpleasant and it can become a recurring problem if you do not treat it effectively. More common in younger women, acute cystitis has a sudden onset with urinary frequency and urgency, and lower abdominal pain being classic symptoms. You need to treat it promptly until symptoms clear, if necessary with antibiotics. Good hydration and good hygiene are essential. Cystitis can also become an ongoing problem, where acute symptoms recur at moments of stress and weakened immune resistance. As tissue in the urinary tract gets progressively weaker, this can lead over time to a chronic form of cystitis and urethritis (see p. 128).

TREATMENT

Start treatment of acute cystitis as soon as you become aware of signs of impending infection. The earlier that you can start herbal treatment, the better the chances of flushing out the infection and avoiding the need for antibiotics. Note: If there is no improvement after three days of treatment, seek professional advice.

+ Pure, unsweetened *cranberry* juice or dried powder (better) is valuable in all urinary tract infections. It works by making it more difficult for bacteria to adhere to the inner lining of the bladder and urinary tubules. *Carrot* juice also works in this way. Take up to 100 ml (3½ fl oz) of juice diluted with water up to three times a day, or take powder as recommended.

+ *Bearberry* and *buchu* are both strong urinary tract disinfectants. Take 20 drops of tincture of either one to five times a day for up to seven days.

+ **To help support the urinary tubules and flush out infection** Take a *cornsilk*, fennel seed, meadowsweet, and/or nettle infusion. Make this using 25 g (1 oz) of a single dried herb or herbs in equal parts to 500 ml (18 fl oz) water a day. *Cornsilk* is the best option when taking a single herb.

+ **To increase the chances of rapid clearance of bacterial infection in more severe cases** Take 2.5 ml (½ tsp) of barberry, marigold, echinacea, or olive leaf once or twice a day. A good combination would be 2.5 ml (½ tsp) of barberry, marigold, and olive leaf tincture in equal parts, taken two to five times a day for up to seven days. (These antimicrobial herbs are not needed in mild cystitis.)

+ Eat a few garlic cloves a day.

CHRONIC CYSTITIS AND URETHRITIS

Chronic cystitis and urethritis are likely to be due to chronic inflammation or a fungal infection, typically *Candida albicans*. These can be difficult problems to treat and may benefit most from professional herbal treatment. That being said, self-help approaches can lead to major improvement. The aim here is to work on several levels to counter infection and inflammation and to strengthen resistance in affected tissue within the urinary tract. Most of the advice given for Acute Cystitis (see p. 127) is directly relevant, and you should consider this first.

TREATMENT	+ Take a *cornsilk*, fennel seed, horsetail, meadowsweet, and/or nettle infusion (see Acute Cytitis). + **To counter underlying infection and strengthen local immune function** Take barberry, *buchu*, marigold, echinacea, and olive leaf tincture. These are best taken in combination, for example: 5 ml (1 tsp) of *buchu* (half part), marigold (two parts), echinacea (two parts) taken two to three times a day.
ADDITIONAL MEASURES	Many other herbs can have a supporting role in relieving symptoms. + **To support tissue repair and for anti-inflammatory activity** Take up to 25 ml (1½ tbsp) of aloe vera juice a day. + **For bladder health** Take 2.5 ml (½ tsp) of horsetail tincture twice a day or take as an infusion using 10 g (⅓ oz) herb to 200 ml (7 fl oz) water. + **To control inflammation within the urinary tract** Take saw palmetto as a concentrated extract.
FROM THE GARDEN	+ Nettle

URINARY FREQUENCY

This intrusive problem can seriously undermine normal life during the day and good quality sleep at night. Several herbs can prove helpful here, soothing bladder irritability. It is not generally a good policy to restrict water intake – for night-time problems, try to drink more in the first half of the day. Avoid alcohol and caffeine.

TREATMENT

+ Take up to 100 ml (3 ½ fl oz) of diluted *cranberry* juice up to three times a day.
+ Take a horsetail infusion. Make it using 10 g (⅓ oz) dried herb to 200 ml (7 fl oz) water. Take 2.5 ml (½ tsp) of horsetail tincture twice a day.
+ Take saw palmetto as a concentrated extract.
+ Take 2.5 ml (½ tsp) of nettle root tincture one to three times a day or take nettle root as a concentrated extract.
+ **For night-time frequency, and especially where anxiety is factor** Take calming remedies, such as passion flower. See Sleep, p. 136.

A COMBINED TREATMENT

Take *cranberry* juice, saw palmetto as a concentrated extract, and 5 ml (1 tsp) of combined horsetail and nettle root tincture (equal parts) three times a day.

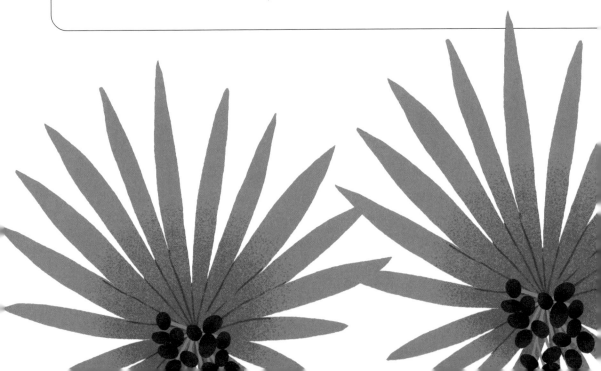

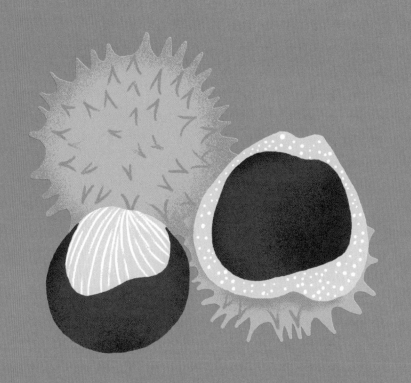

FLUID RETENTION

Being prone to fluid retention, leading to puffy ankles or more system-wide "boggy" skin, causes extra work for the body. A simple approach is to improve flow within the capillary bed and lymphatic network, to allow excess fluid to drain more effectively from the tissues back into the circulation. Treatment needs to be patient and ongoing. If breathlessness or chest pain accompany fluid retention, seek urgent medical advice.

TREATMENT

+ **To stimulate removal of excess fluid** Take a dandelion leaf infusion. Make it using 5–10 g (2½–5 tsp) dried herb to 200 ml (7 fl oz) water. Or take 2.5 ml (½ tsp) of dandelion leaf tincture one to three times a day. Or take a horsetail infusion. Make it using 10 g (⅓ oz) dried herb to 200 ml (7 fl oz) water. Or take 2.5 ml (½ tsp) of horsetail tincture once or twice a day. Or take a nettle infusion. Make it using 10 g (⅓ oz) dried herb to 200 ml (7 fl oz) water. Or take 2.5 ml (½ tsp) of nettle tincture one to three times a day. These remedies are best taken combined in equal parts as an infusion or as 5 ml (1 tsp) of tincture taken two to three times a day.
+ **To support capillary health** Take *bilberry*, *grapeseed*, or *green tea* as concentrated extracts. Take horse chestnut as a concentrated extract. Increase ginger in the diet.

KIDNEY HEALTH

You can safely take several herbs to support kidney function and to slow or prevent the steady deterioration in function that is wrongly seen as inevitable. It is beyond the scope of this book to give specific advice on herbal approaches to treating kidney disease.

TREATMENT

+ Take artichoke as a concentrated extract.
+ Take turmeric as a concentrated extract.
+ Take 2.5 ml (½ tsp) of *astragalus* tincture once or twice a day.
+ Take 2 g (½ tsp) ground milk thistle seeds or take milk thistle as a concentrated extract.
+ Take *bilberry*, *grapeseed*, or *green tea* as concentrated extracts.

Emotional Health

Worry, anxiety, frustration, anger, and irritability are emotions that we experience all too often. When such emotions get stuck, we begin to feel prisoners of them, and they slowly undermine health and well-being – ours, and that of those around us. It would be foolish to think that a herbal remedy or two is going to stop such feelings in their tracks but when chosen well, herbal remedies can make a crucial difference to how you feel. Not giving in and trying out some of these herbs may help you find a way through to a more positive emotional outlook and keep you physically healthy – poor emotional health eventually leads to poor physical health. If the main problem is ongoing stress and exhaustion, see Nervous Exhaustion, p. 89. (See also, Chapter 3: Self Care and Healing).

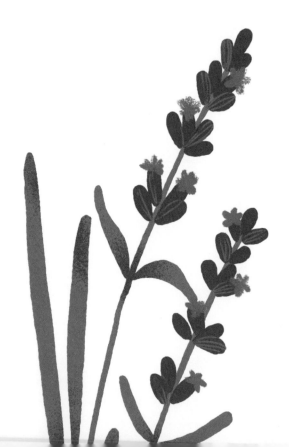

LOW MOOD

Lowered mood, anxiety, and depression are normal after significant emotional loss or separation, and most of us experience lowered mood repeatedly at different times throughout life. Depression can also result from the nervous exhaustion that develops over time with ongoing stress and anxiety. Taking appropriate herbal medicines when you are feeling low or consistently miserable will help to lift your mood and provide greater emotional resilience. St John's wort, the most researched herb for lowered mood and depression is a sensible starting point. With luck, as with lemon balm – described here by Gerard in his *Herbal* (1598) – the following remedies will "comfort the heart, and drive away all melancholy and sadness".

TREATMENT	+ Take 2.5 ml (½ tsp) of St John's wort tincture two to three times a day, or take St John's wort as a concentrated extract for two to three months or more. It can take up to 14 days for positive effects to show through. Caution: You can combine St John's wort with other herbs, but talk with your healthcare practitioner before taking it if you are taking prescribed medication, especially antidepressants.
	+ **Nervous exhaustion** Take 10 saffron strands in food or drink a day. The herb has nerve restorative and protective activity.
	+ **Lowered mood and mild to moderate depression** Take lavender, lemon balm, or rosemary singly or combined as an infusion. Make it using 10 g (⅓ oz) dried herb to 200 ml (7 fl oz) water. Take 2.5 ml (½ tsp) of lavender, lemon balm, or rosemary tincture two to four times a day. If combining tinctures, take 2.5 ml (½ tsp) two to six times a day. All three herbs have neuro-protective activity.
	+ **Low physical and emotional resilience** Take up to 6 g (1 tsp) of ashwagandha powder a day. Take Korean ginseng as a concentrated extract. Take *rhodiola* as a concentrated extract.
FROM THE GARDEN	+ Lavender, lemon balm, rosemary

ANXIETY AND STRESS

While anxiety can be helpful, enabling us to focus on troubles, it is often dysfunctional and creates a state where we feel separated from ourselves and unable to access our natural talents and abilities. Deprived of the ability to engage constructively with life, we feel helpless and experience the unpleasant emotional and physical symptoms that accompany anxiety. Anxiety can also give rise to panic, where the sense of loss of control becomes overwhelming. Herbal remedies rarely provide instant relief in such situations but with a little perseverance they can help you move towards a calmer, more focused state that in turn enables you to map out a route back towards emotional health.

TREATMENT	+ Take a chamomile, lavender, lemon balm, *lime flower*, passion flower, or valerian infusion. Make it using 5–10 g (2½–5 tsp) dried herb to 200 ml (7 fl oz) water.
	+ Take 2.5 ml (½ tsp) of chamomile, lavender, lemon balm, *lime flower*, passion flower, or valerian tincture up to five times a day. If combining herbs, take 2.5 ml (½ tsp) up to eight times a day. A combination of two to three herbs is often best.
	+ Any of the listed herbs can also be taken as concentrated extracts. Take for at least one month.
ADDITIONAL MEASURES	+ To help with poor sleep, palpitations, and ongoing stress, a careful self-assessment might lead to taking passion flower as a concentrated extract, a lemon balm infusion that you make using 10 g (⅓ oz) dried herb to 200 ml (7 fl oz) water per day, and taking ashwagandha as a concentrated extract.
ADDITIONAL SYMPTOMS	Select other herbs to treat the varied symptoms that come with anxiety – headache, poor memory and concentration, restless sleep, digestive disturbance, and palpitations, as well as emotional pressure and distress. For each of these symptoms, it is best to read the relevant sections of this book. Then you will be in a better position to choose appropriate herbs to relieve physical symptoms, to aid relaxation, and to start the process of rebuilding energy reserves.

IRRITABILITY AND ANGER

In traditional herbal medicine, irritability, depression, and anger result from disturbed liver and pancreatic function. In English, to be "liverish" or "bilious" is to be short-tempered and over-reactive, both signs of what would be called "liver-fire" in traditional Chinese medicine. Calming the liver by eating regular meals, avoiding junk food, and by taking herbs that support the liver and pancreas is likely to make you better tempered and less reactive. Add in herbs that relax and enhance vitality, and irritability and anger will become easier to control. See also, Poor Memory and Concentration, p. 90.

TREATMENT

+ **To calm the mind and ease irritability** Take 2.5 ml (½ tsp) of lavender, *lime flower*, passion flower, St John's wort, or valerian tincture as a single herb one to four times a day. To take several in combination, take 5 ml (1 tsp) of tincture in equal parts one to three times a day.
+ **To help support nervous and adrenal gland function** Take the following tonics and adaptogens: up to 6 g (1 tsp) of ashwagandha powder or take ashwagandha as a concentrated extract; 20 drops of liquorice tincture once or twice a day; a sprig of fresh rosemary leaves or 2.5 ml (½ tsp) of rosemary tincture one to three times a day; 2.5 ml (½ tsp) of sage tincture once or twice a day.
+ **For general liver and pancreas support** Take artichoke as a concentrated extract. Take 2 g (½ tsp) of ground milk thistle seed, or take as milk thistle a concentrated extract.

FROM THE GARDEN

+ Lavender, rosemary, sage

Sleep

Regular sleep is something that we take for granted until it is no longer there, like clean air and water. Then we realize how essential it is to life and good health. Occasional, mild sleep disturbance is normal and not a cause for worry. Simple adjustments to your sleep routine – earlier nights, no screen use after a set time, avoiding caffeine after midday – can be sufficient to restore a regular sleep pattern. More chronic sleep problems can be hugely frustrating and require greater attention to sleep routines. In both cases, herbal medicines can help improve sleep quality and duration.

TREATMENT	For occasional difficulty in getting off to sleep:

+ Take 5 ml (1 tsp) of cramp bark, lemon balm, *lime flower*, passion flower, *scullcap*, or valerian tincture, either singly or in combination, once or twice a night. Take a concentrated extract formulated with several of these herbs.
+ **To soothe and relax** Place a few drops of lavender essential oil on your pillow. Place a hop "pillow", a sachet filled with dried hops, next to your pillow.

To reduce waking through the night:

+ Take chaste berry, St John's wort, or valerian as concentrated extracts. Chaste berry raises melatonin levels, St John's wort helps sleep problems linked to depression, and valerian works more on easing anxiety.
+ **To improve sleep quality** Take up to 6 g (1 tsp) of ashwagandha powder. Take ashwagandha, Korean ginseng, or *rhodiola* as concentrated extracts. All three increase the chances of waking in a refreshed state.

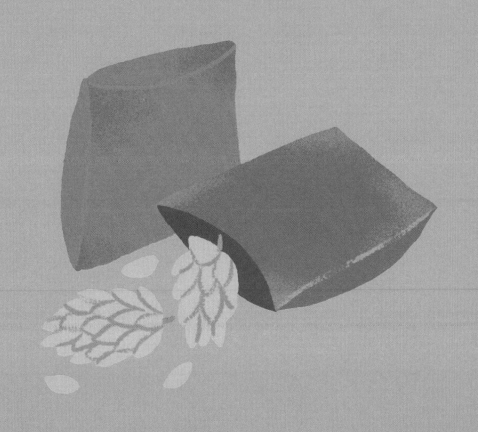

Women's Health

MENSTRUAL PROBLEMS

Women have been using herbs to treat menstrual problems since the earliest times. As a species, we have evolved alongside plants that contain compounds, such as phytoestrogens, which are similar – in some cases identical – to our body's own hormones. Herbal medicine makes use of extracts of these plants to provide subtle, hormonal "nudges" that support the body in regulating and maintaining a symptom-free menstrual cycle. Though professional advice is needed in problems such as polycystic ovary syndrome (PCOS), a self-help approach can heal and rebalance most common menstrual problems.

PRE-MENSTRUAL SYMPTOMS

Pre-menstrual symptoms are a sign of hormonal imbalance, and a fine-tuning of hormone release through the menstrual cycle is essential. However, in order to maintain hormonal balance, hormones need to reach and activate their target cells and the liver needs subsequently to break them down efficiently. Many factors, including congested blood flow, poor liver function, and chronic constipation can interfere in this process, blocking effective communication between the ovaries and womb. The best remedies for pre-menstrual symptoms tend to be gentle hormonal tonics and circulatory stimulants. These will help to improve menstrual regularity, where bleeds are irregular or absent. It usually takes two to three months of taking such remedies before clear-cut signs of improvement begin to show.

+ **Hormonal imbalance** Take 20–40 drops of chaste tree tincture or take chaste tree as a concentrated extract. It is best to take this go-to herb for PMS on waking each morning.

+ **To help strengthen circulation and support liver health** Take 2.5 ml (½ tsp) angelica root or Chinese angelica tincture twice a day. Consume fresh ginger root with food. Eat a sprig of fresh rosemary leaves or take 2.5 ml (½ tsp) of rosemary tincture twice a day. These are all warming tonic herbs. Caution: Do not take angelica or Chinese angelica if you have heavy menstrual bleeding.

+ **Pre-menstrual tension** Take a chamomile infusion. Make it using 10 g (⅓ oz) dried herb to 200 ml (7 fl oz) water. Or take 2.5 ml (½ tsp) of chamomile tincture two to four times a day. Or take a lemon balm infusion. Make it using 10 g (⅓ oz) dried herb to 200 ml (7 fl oz) water. Or take 2.5 ml (½ tsp) of lemon balm tincture two to four times a day. Or take 2.5 ml (½ tsp) of lavender tincture twice a day. These are all relaxant herbs.

+ **Constipation** Chia seeds, flaxseeds, and 5 ml (1 tsp) of dandelion root tincture once or twice a day will be useful. See also, Constipation, p. 117.

+ *Evening primrose* oil capsules can be a valuable supplement for PMS, including breast tenderness and cramps.

FROM THE GARDEN

+ Chamomile, dandelion root, lavender, rosemary

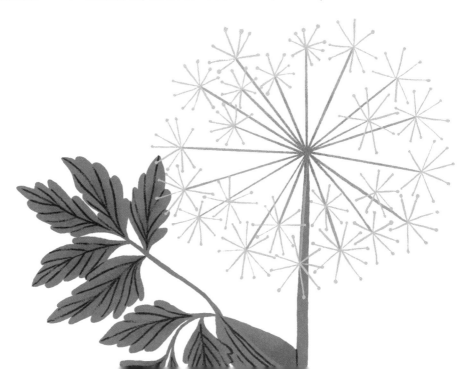

MENSTRUAL CRAMPS AND PAIN

Several herbs provide first-aid relief for menstrual cramps and pain. For best results, start treatment at the first hint of cramps. Cramping muscle pain usually responds well to antispasmodic herbs, such as chamomile and cramp bark. It may be better to treat constant pain with anti-inflammatory remedies such as ginger and turmeric.

TREATMENT	+ **Cramps** Take a chamomile infusion. Make it using 10 g (⅓ oz) dried herb to 200 ml (7 fl oz) water. Or take 2.5 ml (½ tsp) of chamomile tincture two to five times a day. Or take a thyme infusion. Make it using 5 g (2½ tsp) dried herb to 200 ml (7 fl oz) water. Or take 2.5 ml (½ tsp) of thyme tincture two to three times a day. Or take 5 ml (1 tsp) of cramp bark tincture up to five times a day. Singly or in combination, these herbs should bring quick relief.
	+ **For pain relief** Take 2.5 ml (½ tsp) of black cohosh tincture once or twice a day. Or take 2.5 ml (½ tsp) of lavender tincture once or twice a day. Or take 2.5 ml (½ tsp) of valerian tincture one to four times a day or take valerian as a concentrated extract. Massage lavender essential oil into the abdomen.
	+ As anti-inflammatories, eat fresh ginger root or take ginger as a concentrated extract. Take turmeric as a concentrated extract (a low dose throughout the month and a higher dose at the onset of pain).
FROM THE GARDEN	+ Chamomile, lavender, thyme

AN EFFECTIVE COMBINATION	Take 5 ml (1 tsp) of black cohosh (one part), chamomile (two parts), valerian (two parts) tincture up to five times a day for up to one week. A standard dose is 5 ml (1 tsp) one to three times a day.

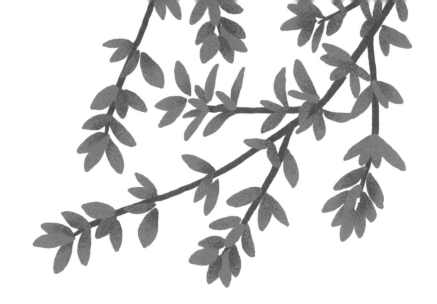

HEAVY MENSTRUAL BLEEDING

Heavy menstrual bleeding is linked to low progesterone and excess oestrogen release by the ovaries. This leads to increased growth of the lining of the womb prior to menstruation, causing clotting, heavy bleeding, and over several months can lead to anaemia and low iron reserves. Suggested Remedies support balanced hormone levels through the cycle, control bleeding, and promote vitality.

TREATMENT	+ Take chaste berry tincture, see Pre-Menstrual Symptoms, p. 138. + **To control bleeding** Take a nettle leaf infusion. Make it using 10–15 g (⅓–½ oz) dried herb to 200 ml (7 fl oz) water. Or take 5 ml (1 tsp) of nettle tincture three to four times a day. Or take a *raspberry leaf* infusion. Make it using 10 g (⅓ oz) dried herb to 200 ml (7 fl oz) water. Or take 2.5 ml (½ tsp) of *yarrow* tincture twice a day. You can take these three herbs in combination. + **For anaemia, chronic stress, and overwork** Take up to 6 g (1 tsp) of ashwagandha powder a day. Take 2.5–5 g (½–1 tsp) of dried nettle seed or powder a day. Take 2.5–5 g (½–1 tsp) of maca powder a day.
FROM THE GARDEN	+ Nettle leaf and seed

VAGINAL HEALTH

In good vaginal health, secretions from the mucous membranes of
the vaginal wall maintain a steady acidic environment (pH 3.5–4.5),
making the vagina a relatively hostile place for potential pathogens – a
key factor in preventing vaginal infection and inflammation. The low pH
also encourages a healthy, stable bacterial population within the vagina,
which supports mucous membrane health and resilience. Adequate
oestrogen levels are also essential for good vaginal health, particularly
from the menopause onwards. Used carefully, herbal remedies can be
very effective in treating vaginal symptoms and promoting better bacterial
and hormonal balance.

DISCOMFORT AND ITCHING

Discomfort and itching is usually a sign of mild fungal irritation. You can
relieve symptoms using a few simple remedies. For candida, see Vaginal
Infection, p. 144.

TREATMENT	+ Apply aloe vera gel or juice, marigold or chamomile cream, or *coconut* oil. Add a drop or two of lavender, *geranium*, or *tea tree* essential oil per 5 ml (1 tsp) cream or oil. + Take a marigold infusion. Make it using 10 g (⅓ oz) to 200 ml (7 fl oz) water. + Take 2.5 ml (½ tsp) of olive leaf tincture two to three times a day.
FROM THE GARDEN	+ Marigold, chamomile

DRYNESS, SORENESS, AND INFLAMMATION

Mild-acting, hormonal plant extracts and soothing demulcent remedies will often make a major difference to these conditions.

TREATMENT	+ Take chaste berry tincture, a herb for low progesterone levels, see Pre-Menstrual Symptoms, p. 138. + Take 2.5 ml (½ tsp) of black cohosh tincture, once or twice a day, 2.5 ml (½ tsp) of fennel seed tincture, once or twice a day, or 2.5 ml (½ tsp) of *shatavari* tincture one to three times a day. These tonic herbs have oestrogenic activity and help to strengthen vaginal tissue. As a combined tincture take 5 ml (1 tsp) one to three times a day. + Take 10–20 g (⅓–¾ oz) of ground chia seeds or flaxseeds a day. + **To soothe, counter inflammation, and support healing of the vaginal wall** Apply chamomile cream or carefully blend 10 drops each of *fenugreek* and liquorice tincture (or 20 drops of just one herb) per 10 ml (2 tsp) of chamomile cream. Apply one to three times a day.
FROM THE GARDEN	+ Chamomile

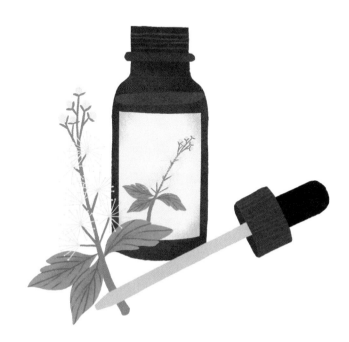

VAGINAL INFECTION

Mild infections respond well to herbal remedies and they often clear quickly. Start treatment as soon as symptoms appear. Bacterial and fungal infections require slightly different approaches (see also, Candida Infection, below). Where cystitis-type symptoms are present, take *cranberry* extract and refer to Cystitis, p. 127. In instances of significant pain or non-menstrual bleeding, seek professional advice.

TREATMENT

+ **For quick relief** Add 5 ml (1 tsp) of propolis tincture to 100 ml (3½ fl oz) warm water and use as a vaginal wash. Caution: If you have never used propolis tincture before, test it on your skin first.
+ Apply marigold or chamomile cream, blended with 15 drops of liquorice tincture and 15 drops of *goldenseal* tincture per 10 ml (2 tsp) of cream. For bacterial infection, add in two drops of *geranium* or *tea tree* essential oil per 10 ml (2 tsp) of cream. Apply small amounts of cream frequently.
+ **To counter infection and stimulate local immune resistance** Take 5 ml (1 tsp) of barberry (one part), marigold (two parts), echinacea (two parts), and olive leaf (two parts) combined tincture two to three times a day.

CANDIDA INFECTION

All the above suggestions are useful when treating fungal infection, especially candidiasis. There are also a few additional remedies that act specifically against candida.

TREATMENT

+ Add 2 drops of *clove* or thyme essential oil per 10 ml (2 tsp) of marigold or chamomile cream.
+ Make a turmeric infusion made by steeping 20 g (¾ oz) powder to 200 ml (7 fl oz) water for 10 minutes. Strain thoroughly, cool to body temperature, and apply as a vaginal wash.
+ Take *pau d'arco* as a concentrated extract. Caution: Do not take *pau d'arco* if you are pregnant.

FROM THE GARDEN

+ Marigold, chamomile, echinacea, thyme

PREGNANCY AND BREASTFEEDING

Herbal remedies are safe to take during pregnancy, though for the first three months of pregnancy take herbs only on professional advice (using herbs and spices in cooking is fine). From four months onwards, you can use a range of safe and effective remedies to treat simple health problems such as colds, catarrh, and constipation. Look up the recommended treatment – for example, for Nausea and Vomiting, p. 113 – but only select remedies from the list of safe herbs to use on the following pages, all of which are known to be mild acting and safe during pregnancy and while breastfeeding.

If taking manufactured remedies, check the labels carefully, especially where herbs and other constituents are combined. Take infusions, powders, or tablets in preference to tinctures, which contain alcohol. Alcohol should be avoided during the first three months of pregnancy, even in the small amounts present in tinctures.

When using the herbs suggested in remedies, check the advice given for each one and stick to the recommended dosages. Some of the herbs listed in Chapter 5 – for example, barberry and sage – are known to be unsafe during pregnancy, as they can cause miscarriage: do not take them. You will find lists of herbs that are safe to use and not safe to use during pregnancy and while breastfeeding on page 147.

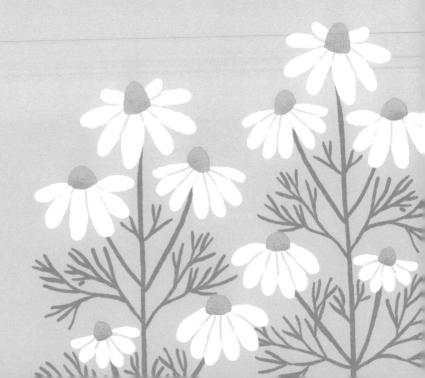

PREPARING FOR CHILDBIRTH

Raspberry leaf is the safest and most researched herb used to prepare for childbirth. Those who use it take it during the last trimester, when it is thought to relax the muscles of the cervix and tone up the long muscles of the womb that push the baby out. Iranian research indicates that *date* fruit can also help prepare for childbirth – eat *dates* from week thirty-six.

TREATMENT

+ Take a *raspberry leaf* infusion. Make it using 5–10 g (2½–5 tsp) dried herb or a *raspberry leaf* teabag to 200 ml (7 fl oz) water. Take 4–8 g (½–1½ tsp) *raspberry* leaf powder a day. Take *raspberry leaf* as a concentrated extract. Take a higher dose towards the end of your pregnancy.
+ Eat 3–4 *medjool dates* a day.

BREASTFEEDING

Herbal remedies can prove very useful during breastfeeding. Take them as needed to improve the flow of breast milk or to help relieve discomfort and engorgement. They also make a useful aid to weaning. All the remedies suggested here are safe and known to be helpful. Many seeds stimulate the production and flow of breast milk.

TREATMENT

+ **To increase milk flow** Take 1 g (½ tsp) of fennel seeds, *fenugreek* seeds, or milk thistle seeds once a day. Up the dosage to twice a day if needed. Other herbs to try include garlic and ginger, which can be used in cooking.
+ **To reduce breast milk and to aid weaning** Take a peppermint, rosemary, or sage infusion. Make it using 5 g (2½ tsp) dried herb or a teabag to 200 ml (7 fl oz) water and drink it throughout the day.
+ **Engorgement and breast tenderness** Massage marigold or chamomile cream into tender areas. Both are also good for sore and cracked nipples. Take a marigold infusion. Make it using 10 g (⅓ oz) dried herb to 200 ml (7 fl oz) water. Take 2.5 ml (½ tsp) of marigold tincture one to three times a day. Make a *marshmallow* leaf infusion using 5–15 g (2½–5 tsp) dried herb to 200 ml (7 fl oz) water. Steep it for 15 minutes and use the warm leaves to make a compress or soak a cloth in the warm liquid and apply to your breasts.

SAFE HERBS TO USE DURING PREGNANCY AND WHILE BREASTFEEDING

+ Marigold
+ Chamomile
+ Chia seed
+ *Cornsilk*
+ Cramp bark
+ Dandelion
+ Echinacea
+ Elderflower and berry
+ Flaxseed
+ Garlic
+ Ginger
+ Lavender

+ Lemon balm
+ *Lime flower*
+ Milk thistle
+ Nettle
+ Passion flower
+ Peppermint
+ *Raspberry leaf*
+ *Rhubarb root*
+ *Senna*
+ Turmeric
+ Valerian

HERBS THAT ARE *NOT* SAFE TO USE DURING PREGNANCY OR WHILE BREASTFEEDING

+ Angelica
+ Chinese angelica
+ Barberry
+ Black cohosh
+ Saffron
+ Liquorice
+ Elecampane

+ Korean ginseng
+ Sage
+ Saw palmetto
+ Chaste tree
+ Ashwagandha

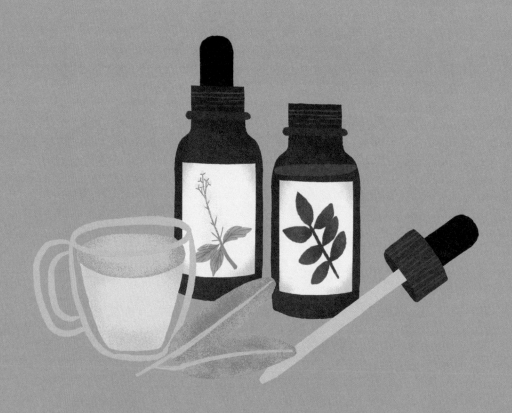

MENOPAUSE

A herbal approach to the menopause aims to support oestrogen levels and aid the body in adapting successfully to a new hormonal balance. Many oestrogenic and tonic herbs will help in this process and relieve menopausal symptoms. Other factors common in mid-life, such as raised stress levels, reduced vitality, and poor sleep, can be factors contributing to menopausal symptoms and, in fact, hot flushing and vaginal dryness are thought to be the only menopausal symptoms due solely to low oestrogen levels. As ovarian oestrogen production declines, so the adrenal glands and body fat tissue compensate by releasing higher (though still small) levels of oestrogen. Supporting adrenal gland health – essential for vitality and well-being – can also help to minimize symptoms associated with the menopause. Reviewing your health as a whole and then using a combination of hormonal and restorative/tonic herbs can make a notable difference at the menopause. For vaginal dryness and discomfort, see Vaginal Health, p. 142 and for lowered mood and vitality, see Low Mood, p. 133 and Nervous Exhaustion p. 89.

POOR MENTAL FOCUS

Loss of mental sharpness and a poorly functioning memory are common problems during the menopause. Herbal medicines can prove extremely useful in reversing and restoring normal cognition. The herbs listed below promote circulation to the brain and/or have neuroprotective activity. See also, Poor Memory and Cognition, p. 90.

TREATMENT
+ Take 2.5 ml (½ tsp) of Chinese angelica tincture once or twice a day.
+ Take ginkgo as a concentrated extract.
+ Take a lemon balm infusion. Make it using 10 g (⅓ oz) dried herb to 200 ml (7 fl oz) water. Take 5 ml (1 tsp) of lemon balm tincture once or twice a day.
+ Eat a sprig of fresh rosemary fresh leaves or take 2.5 ml (½ tsp) of rosemary tincture once or twice a day.
+ Take 2.5 ml (½ tsp) of sage tincture once or twice a day.
+ Eat 10 saffron filaments a day and take *bilberry*, *grapeseed*, or *green tea* as concentrated extracts.
+ For best results, take several herbs together, for example, ginkgo as a concentrated extract and lemon balm tincture.

SUPPORTING LIBIDO

Many herbs are known to enhance libido and vitality – perhaps the foremost being *shatavari*, known in India as the "Queen of Herbs". A nourishing oestrogenic herb, *shatavari* maintains health and well-being, encourages sexual desire, and works well as short- or long-term as a menopausal tonic. The other herbs listed can be equally helpful.

TREATMENT

+ Take 3–10 g (½–2 tsp) of *shatavari* powder a day or take *shatavari* as a concentrated extract.
+ Take up to 6 g (1 tsp) of ashwagandha powder a day or 5 ml (1 tsp) of ashwagandha tincture once or twice a day.
+ Take 2.5 ml (½ tsp) of Chinese angelica tincture once or twice a day.
+ Take 2–4 g (½–1 tsp) of maca powder a day.

DISTURBED SLEEP AND NIGHT SWEATS

See Sleep, p. 136, for detailed advice on herbal medicines to promote better sleep. The following additional suggestions are aimed at reducing the frequency and intensity of sweats and flushing at night.

TREATMENT

+ **For night sweats** Take 20 drops of sage tincture up to four times a night (maximum 80 drops a day).
+ **To improve sleep quality and reduce night sweats** Take 2.5 ml (½ tsp) of St John's wort tincture once or twice at night (maximum 5 ml/1 tsp a day). Take St John's wort as a concentrated extract.
+ Take *hops* as a concentrated extract in combination with herbs such as valerian. *Hops* are oestrogenic, cooling and sedative, in theory making them an ideal remedy for sleep broken by night sweats. A hop pillow can be a boon.

HOT FLUSHING AND SWEATS

Women have long used herbs to relieve hot flushing and sweats. In the UK, sage tea is the main traditional remedy for these problems, in North America it is black cohosh, and in Russia, liquorice. Research indicates that all three are indeed valuable remedies for menopausal symptoms.

TREATMENT

+ **To control sweats** Take a sage infusion. Make it using 5 g (2½ tsp) dried herb to 200 ml (7 fl oz) water.
+ **For lowered mood and emotional exhaustion** Take 2.5 ml (½ tsp) black cohosh tincture once or twice a day. Take with 2.5 ml (½ tsp) of St John's wort tincture one to three times a day or take black cohosh and St John's wort combined as concentrated extracts.
+ **For adrenal gland support** Take 20 drops of liquorice tincture one to three times a day or take liquorice as a concentrated extract.
+ **To restore adrenal gland function and promote vitality** Take up to 6 g (1 tsp) of ashwagandha powder a day. Take ashwagandha or Korean ginseng as concentrated extracts. Take 2–4 g (½–1 tsp) of maca powder a day.
+ Valuable supplements include chia seeds and flaxseeds, both of which contain phytoestrogens and omega-3 oils.

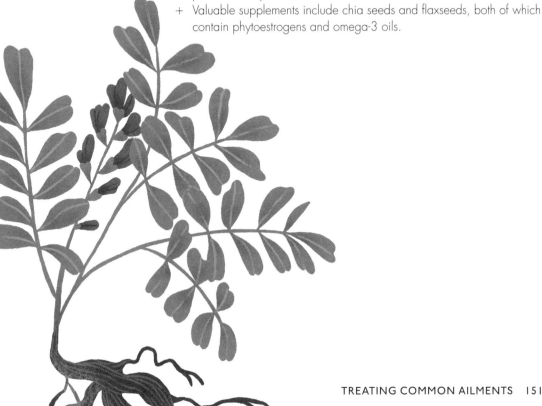

Men's Health

In men, an enlarged prostate and difficulty passing urine become increasingly common with age and are often associated with loss of libido and erectile dysfunction. Such conditions generally cause discomfort and a sense of embarrassment, though poor bladder emptying and concerns about prostate cancer are issues that can have a greater impact in the long-term. Herbal medicine has a history of helping to prevent and heal these conditions, though treatment works best if started in the early stages of symptoms.

PROSTATE HEALTH

Benign prostatic hypertrophy (BPH) and infection of the prostate (prostatitis) are common problems, especially in later years, and often occur together. Several herbs, notably saw palmetto, are effective in treating BPH and will often relieve symptoms after a few weeks. Where symptoms do not respond in this way, treating possible underlying prostate infection and inflammation may help. Lycopene-rich foods, such as tomatoes and watermelon, and pumpkin seeds (1–2 handfuls a day) support prostate health.

TREATMENT

+ Take saw palmetto as a concentrated extract.
+ Take a nettle root decoction. Make it using 10 g (⅓ oz) dried herb to 200 ml (7 fl oz) water. Take 5 ml (1 tsp) of nettle root tincture once or twice a day.
+ Take a *small-leaved willowherb* infusion. Make it using 2.5–5 g (2½–5 tsp) dried herb to 200 ml (7 fl oz) water. Take 2.5 ml (½ tsp) of *small-leaved willowherb* tincture once or twice a day.
+ Apply aloe vera, horse chestnut, or witch hazel lotion or cream onto the skin overlying the prostate (the perineum) once or twice a day.
+ Olive leaf tincture and turmeric powder or concentrated extracts are valuable remedies for chronic prostatitis and can be effective additional remedies in BPH.

POOR URINE FLOW AND FREQUENCY

The medical term for these problems is lower urinary tract syndrome (LUTS) and by and large these symptoms reflect bladder irritation and a reduced diameter in the urethra. BPH often accompanies or causes these symptoms, with the prostate pressing on the urethra, increasing the pressure needed to pass urine effectively. When combined with BPH treatment, the following herbs, especially horsetail, will help relieve symptoms. Treatment needs to be long term.

TREATMENT

+ Take *varuna* (*Crataeva nurvula*) as a concentrated extract.
+ Take 2.5 ml (½ tsp) of horsetail tincture one to three times a day.
+ Take a nettle leaf infusion. Make it using 10 g (⅓ oz) dried herb to 200 ml (7 fl oz) water. Take 5 ml (1 tsp) of nettle leaf tincture once or twice a day.

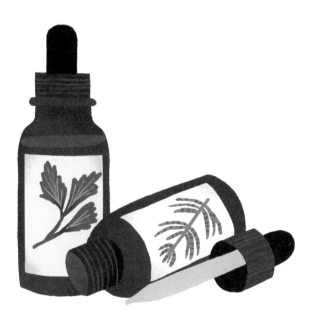

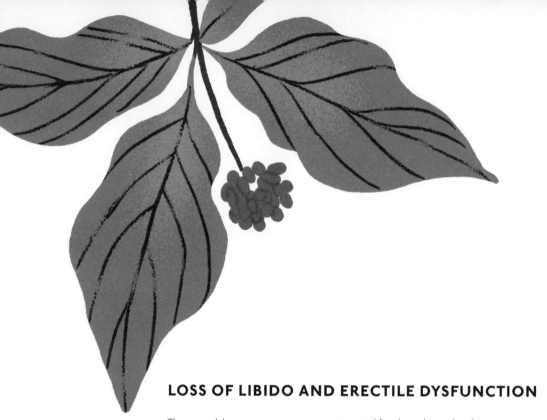

LOSS OF LIBIDO AND ERECTILE DYSFUNCTION

These problems can occur at any time in life, though tend to happen more frequently with age. Several herbs, notably ashwagandha and Korean ginseng, are prized for their ability to enhance libido and resolve sexual dysfunction. Alongside the supportive hormonal activity these adaptogens provide, herbs such as ginkgo that improve blood flow to the penis can be important. Problems involving sexual dysfunction are often entwined within an emotional context, so relaxant herbs like passion flower that calm the sense of needing to perform, may prove helpful.

TREATMENT

+ Take up to 6 g (1 tsp) ashwagandha powder a day or take ashwagandha as a concentrated extract.
+ Take Korean ginseng as a concentrated extract. Take up to 4 g (1 tsp) of maca powder a day. Take *rhodiola* as a concentrated extract.
+ **To improve hormonal balance and raise testosterone levels** Take saw palmetto as a concentrated extract. Take 2.5 ml (½ tsp) of nettle root tincture one to three times a day.
+ **To strengthen local blood flow** Take 2.5 ml (½ tsp) of Chinese angelica tincture twice a day. Take ginger root with food. Take ginkgo as a concentrated extract.

Children's Health

The speed and intensity with which children can become ill – fine on waking, a 40°C (104°F) fever by 10.00 am – can be deeply worrying for parents and carers. Fortunately, children have strong-acting, efficient immune systems, which enables them to recover as speedily as they fall ill – the sick child on waking is running around again four hours later. This means that most ill health in children is short-lasting. Home treatment is about managing symptoms over a relatively short period of time: keeping a fever under control, easing discomfort or pain, soothing fractiousness and irritability, and aiding restful sleep.

The following pages focus on treatment for ailments in babies and young children (six months to six years old). For children aged seven years and older, use treatments recommended in the adult section of this chapter but at the appropriate dosages for their age, see p. 157.

"RED FLAG" SIGNS AND SYMPTOMS	In most cases, you can use herbal treatment safely to relieve symptoms and speed your child's recovery. But if your child's symptoms are severe (see "Red Flag" signs and symptoms, pp. 22–23), or do not follow the expected pattern for your child, you should seek immediate advice from your healthcare practitioner.

HERBS FOR INTERNAL USE

+ *Aniseed*
+ Marigold
+ *Caraway*
+ Chamomile
+ Chia seed
+ Cinnamon*
+ Dandelion
+ Echinacea*
+ Elderflower and berry
+ Elecampane*
+ Fennel
+ Garlic
+ Ginger*
+ *Lime flower*
+ *Marshmallow*
+ Meadowsweet
+ Nettle
+ Passion flower
+ Peppermint*
+ Plantain
+ *Slippery elm*
+ Thyme*
+ Valerian*

*not suitable for children under one

HERBS FOR EXTERNAL USE

+ Aloe vera
+ Arnica
+ Marigold
+ Chamomile
+ *Chickweed*
+ Echinacea
+ Garlic
+ Plantain
+ *Slippery elm*
+ Witch hazel

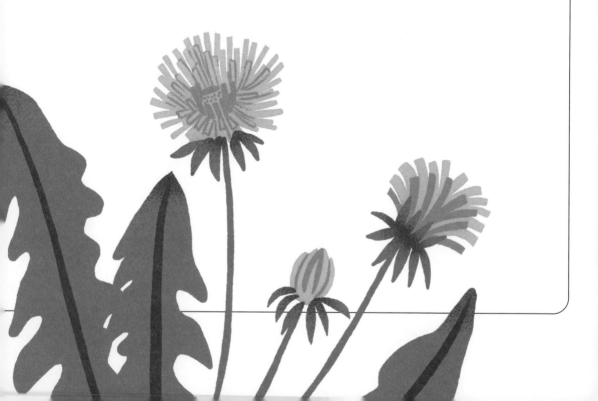

PREPARATIONS SUITABLE FOR CHILDREN

Once you have decided what herb(s) to give your child, the question is, in what form and how much?

+ Infusions and teas are generally best for children as they are diluted and water-based (during a fever, drinking large quantities of water is essential). Infusions can be sweetened with honey, maple syrup, or concentrated *apple* juice. For colds, sore throats, coughs, and chesty conditions, honey makes a valuable addition to infusions (usually 5 ml/1 tsp to 200 ml/7 fl oz) water.
+ You can also use infusions as compresses, lotions, hand or foot baths, and inhalations.
+ Adding an infusion of a gentle-acting herb such as chamomile or marigold to a warm bath is an excellent way to treat young children.
+ Tablets may be hard to swallow and you may need to cut them into halves or quarters to achieve the right dose. You can crush them and mix them with honey.
+ You can add powders or opened capsules to food or drink at the right dose.
+ Tinctures are convenient, but are not suitable for babies and infants as they contain alcohol. To measure small amounts of tincture, put the tincture in a clean dropper bottle and carefully measure out: 1 ml = 20 drops using standard size dropper.

When breastfeeding, the best method is to take the herb(s) for your child, who will then benefit from them through your milk. Take the regular adult dose in this situation.

RECOMMENDED DOSAGES FOR CHILDREN

+ Babies (six to twelve months): ⅒ adult dose
+ Infants (one to three years): ¼ adult dose
+ Young children (five to eight years): ⅓ adult dose
+ Older children (nine to twelve years): ½–⅔ adult dose

Always start with a low dose and build up as required. Children can respond very quickly to herbal medicines. You can adapt a dose up or down for children who are significantly above or below average size for their age.

COLIC

Medicinal herbs are the main ingredients in many over-the-counter remedies for colic and griping pains. Known as gripe waters, these traditional remedies contain the distilled water of herbs such as *aniseed*, *caraway*, and fennel, which gently soothe irritability and cramping within the gut. They are specifically formulated for babies and young children. Self-help remedies prepared at home can be just as safe.

TREATMENT

+ Make a chamomile infusion using a chamomile teabag or 10 g (⅓ oz) dried herb to 200 ml (7 fl oz) water. Give your child tablespoon doses in a bottle or cup.
+ Make a fennel infusion using a fennel teabag or 5 g (2½ tsp) dried herb to 200 ml (7 fl oz) water. Give your child tablespoon doses in a bottle or cup.

COLDS AND CATARRH

These common problems in young children usually respond well to herbal treatment. See Colds and Flu, p. 103 and Sinus Problems and Catarrh, p. 105 for detailed advice. The herbs recommended in these sections are safe for children when taken at the correct dose (see p. 157).

ADDITIONAL TREATMENT

+ Make an elderflower infusion using 10 g (⅓ oz) dried herb to 200 ml (7 fl oz) water. Give your child regular tablespoon doses in a bottle or cup. This is the best remedy for upper respiratory infections and catarrh in babies and children up to their second birthday. A chamomile infusion can also be helpful.
+ Propolis tincture/extract is suitable from age two in very small doses: 1 drop for two to four years; 2–3 drops for children aged five to nine; 10–20 drops for children aged 10 to 12. Always carry out a patch test first.

CRADLE CAP AND SKIN RASHES

Cradle cap is a yeast problem, like dandruff. It is important to brush the hair and scalp daily and to use a simple shampoo for washing the hair. Simple herbal creams and oils can help.

TREATMENT

+ Gently massage marigold cream, *coconut* oil, or olive oil into the affected areas once or twice a day.

HEADLICE

Headlice can be a very troublesome problem and hard to get rid of. The following mild-acting treatments can help.

TREATMENT

+ **Nits** Combine 10 drops of *neem* oil or *tea tree* oil with 25 ml (1 ½ tbsp) *coconut* or olive oil and massage thoroughly into the hair and scalp. Leave it on for one hour, then wash it out.
+ **Lice** Add 1–2 drops of *neem* oil or *tea tree* oil to shampoo.
+ To prevent reinfection, regularly apply *coconut* oil or olive oil to the hair and scalp.

NAPPY RASH

It is best to apply herbs as ointments to treat nappy rash. Being impermeable, they protect the skin from irritation caused by urine. Gels, lotions, and creams support healing but do not protect the skin.

TREATMENT

+ Apply aloe vera, marigold, or chamomile ointment as needed or add 1 drop of *tea tree* oil to 5 ml (1 tsp) ointment and mix thoroughly.

THREADWORM

Home treatment with herbs can be effective for threadworm in children. Treatment using well-tolerated herbs over a four-week period has the best chance of clearing the infestation.

TREATMENT

+ Make a thyme infusion using 2.5 g (1 level tsp) dried herb to 100 ml (3½ fl oz) water. For children up to two years, give up to 15 ml (1 tbsp); for children aged two to four, give up to 30 ml (2 tbsp); for children aged four to six, give up to 60 ml (4 tbsp).
+ Add 5–10 g (1–2 tsp) of ground *pumpkin* seeds a day to food, mixed with honey.
+ Add fresh garlic root to food or give garlic as a concentrated extract.

CONSTIPATION AND DIARRHOEA

Though it may sound unlikely, the best option for both problems is chamomile. Constipation in young children is almost always due to over-contracted muscles in the colon, preventing a normal bowel movement. A chamomile infusion (or distilled water) will usually be sufficient to relax this muscle tension and relieve constipation. For diarrhoea and loose stools, chamomile and meadowsweet are excellent herbs of choice. Make sure your child drinks plenty of liquid to prevent dehydration.

TREATMENT

+ **Constipation** Make a chamomile infusion using a teabag or 10 g (⅓ oz) dried herb to 200 ml (7 fl oz) water. Give this to your child in regular tablespoon doses. Where constipation is an ongoing problem, include 2 g (½–1 tsp) of soaked chia seeds routinely in semi-liquid food, such as porridge or stewed *apples*.
+ **Diarrhoea** Make a chamomile or meadowsweet infusion using a teabag or 10 g (⅓ oz) dried herb to 200 ml (7 fl oz) water. Give this to your child in regular tablespoon doses. A fennel infusion is also good. Meadowsweet is gently astringent, both herbs relieve inflammation within the gut. If diarrhoea occurs regularly, include 2 g (½–1 tsp) of soaked chia seeds in the diet.

SLEEP

The best remedies to aid sleep in children are relaxants that relieve anxiety, irritability, and tension and encourage your child to drift off into a relaxed sleep.

TREATMENT

+ Make a chamomile, passion flower, or Californian poppy infusion using a teabag or 5 g (2½ tsp) dried herb to 200 ml (7 fl oz) water. For children up to two years old, give up to 15 ml (1 tbsp); for children aged two to four, give up to 30 ml (2 tbsp); for children aged four to six, give up to 60 ml (4 tbsp).

TEETHING

An old remedy for teething is a length of *marshmallow* root. The sleep remedies listed below may also be useful.

TREATMENT

+ Give a 5-cm-long (2½ in) piece of *marshmallow* root to your child to chew. As the child chews, the outside of the root quickly becomes gooey and soothing to the gums.
+ Mix chamomile infusion into a paste with *slippery elm* powder and apply to your child's gums.

TEEN HEALTH

You can consult the adult section of this chapter for treating teenagers. Below is a list of typical teen health problems, together with recommended herbs for treating them.

Acne (see p. 73) — Marigold, echinacea, chaste berry
Hair care (see p. 78) — Chamomile, nettle, olive oil
Preparing for exams (see p. 90) — Ginkgo, rosemary, saffron
Respiratory infection (see p. 102) — Echinacea, elderberry, propolis
Lowered mood (see p. 133) — Lemon balm, rosemary, St John's wort
Anxiety and stress (see p. 134) — Lavender, passion flower, valerian
Sleep disturbance (see p. 136) — Ashwagandha, Californian poppy, valerian

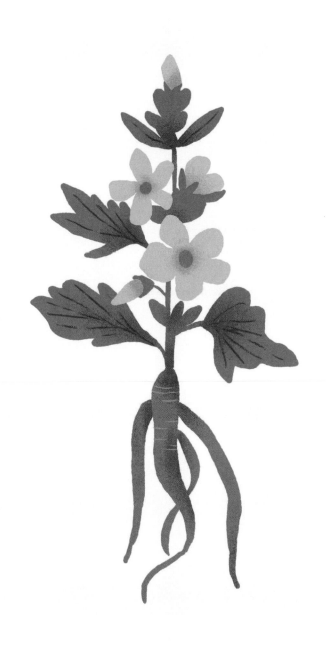

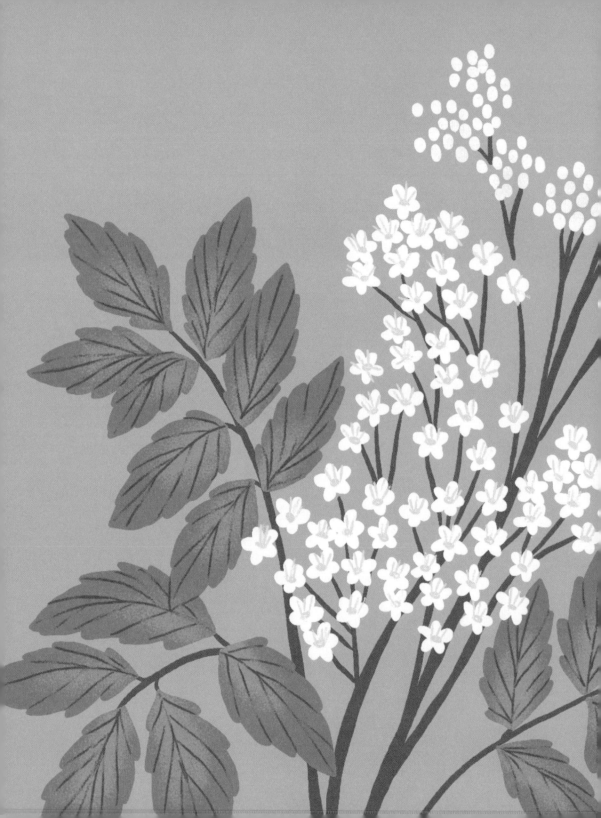

Herb Profiles

This chapter provides detailed profiles of 50 key medicinal plants. Many of them are familiar kitchen remedies. Each entry lists the herb's main actions and therapeutic uses. There are clear recommendations to ensure safe use, including dosage, length of use, cautions, and helpful herb combinations.

5

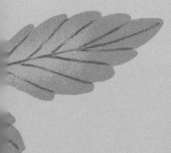

Introduction to the Herb Profiles

From the hundreds of herbs that could have been included in this book, 50 key plants have been selected – not a straightforward task. The herbs have been selected for their usefulness in home treatment, recognized safety and effectiveness, availability in health stores and online, sustainability, the possibility and ease of growing them at home, and cost. You are entirely free to use other herbs as appropriate, though at least to begin with, it is good to stick to a limited number of remedies and to become familiar with using them and discovering how they work in practice.

Each herb profile opens with a short summary of how it is generally used as a remedy. This is followed by a list of the herb's key actions and main uses. Practical advice on how best to take the herb, dosage, and cautions aims to enable you to use the herb in a safe and effective manner. The profile finishes with suggested combinations for specific health complaints. Most of the text is self-explanatory but please bear in mind the following points when reading the entries.

+ The main uses listed are those suitable for self-treatment. Uses that require professional skill and experience are not included.
+ The "best taken as" section lists the types of herbal preparations most likely to prove effective when using the herb. Other preparations may also prove useful – the list does not mean the herb has to be used in this way.
+ Tablets and capsules: so many different products are available for most of the herbs covered that it makes sense to distinguish between simple herbal preparations and concentrated extracts (see A Note on Terminology, p. 167).

A NOTE ON TERMINOLOGY

Simple herbal preparations include fresh or dried herb material that is made up into infusions, decoctions, or tinctures, or taken as a powder or capsule containing unprocessed ground herb material. Specific dosages are given for these preparations. Please see section on dosage pp. 224–225 for further information.

Concentrated extracts are manufactured products, where the herb is industrially processed to concentrate the active constituents. These are usually formulated and sold as tablets, capsules, or liquid extracts. The level of concentration typically varies between one manufacturer and another, so it is not possible to give a standard dose for such concentrated extracts. Follow the manufacturer's recommendations on dosage or seek advice from a herbal practitioner or naturopath, who may on occasions recommend a higher than normal dose.

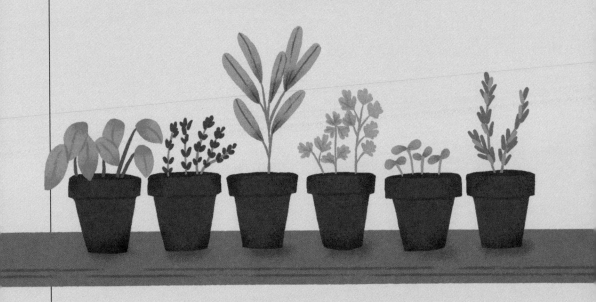

USES AND ACTIONS

At the start of every herb profile in this chapter, there is a list of main uses (also called indications) and main actions for that particular herb. The lists provide a summary of the herb's medicinal uses and therapeutic actions. Understanding a herb's indications is relatively easy – these are the ailments the herb is commonly used for. Understanding a herb's actions is more complex, but is worthwhile in the long-term. Here are the main uses and actions for rosemary:

MAIN USES

Nervous exhaustion, chronic stress, lowered mood, poor memory and cognition, low blood pressure, failure to thrive, weak digestion, dizziness, to reduce the risk of sunburn, to slow the ageing processes.

Looking first at the main uses, this information is enough for you to know the main conditions rosemary will help to treat. The herb is a perfect example of a tonic that supports vitality, mood, and mental function when the body is under-performing or subject to chronic stress. But while knowing the main uses for each herb is useful, it does not give you the ability to choose between different herbs and select those most likely to be of help in a given situation. This is why herbalists focus on a herb's main actions.

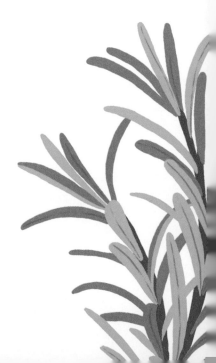

Neuroprotective, mild antidepressant, anti-inflammatory, bitter tonic, circulatory tonic, antiageing, protects against sunburn.

In the example here, rosemary has a wide range of actions that affect the body and mind in different ways:

+ "Neuroprotective" means a herb protects nerve cells from damage, degeneration, and impairment.

+ Add in the herb's anti-inflammatory activity and its ability to improve blood flow to the brain, and it is clear that rosemary is a key herb for brain health.

+ Consider the remaining actions in this way, and you begin to see a complex combination of effects that together make up the unique therapeutic profile of rosemary.

Learning about the actions of herbs in this way brings an extra dimension of understanding to using them as remedies. In time, this will enable you to gain a sense of each herb's special characteristics and to recognize key differences between similar-acting herbs.

Horse chestnut

Aesculus hippocastanum

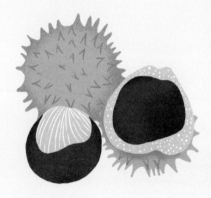

Horse chestnut is well-researched and a key remedy for venous problems. Extracts may be taken safely to treat acute conditions, such as hot and painful haemorrhoids, as well as in longstanding, chronic problems, such as varicose veins and associated swelling. Extracts support the return of fluid into the veins, minimizing the impact of leakage into the surrounding area, when the integrity of a vein is compromised. Extracts also aid repair of distended veins and can, potentially at least, heal varicose veins, if treated early on in their development.

PARTS USED
Seed

MAIN USES
Varicose veins, thread veins, varicose eczema, fluid retention and "boggy" conditions (especially in the legs), restless legs, haemorrhoids, arthritis

MAIN ACTIONS
Vein tonic, circulatory tonic

BEST TAKEN AS
Internal use
+ Tincture, concentrated extracts
External use
+ Lotion or gel

DOSAGE
Internal use
+ Tincture 2.5–5 ml (½–1 tsp) a day
External use
+ Apply lotion/gel as required

LENGTH OF TREATMENT
Can be taken long-term to prevent or treat vein problems. Take for up to three months to see clear improvement in vein problems.

CAUTIONS
Horse chestnut is toxic in excess and can cause nausea, digestive upset, and diarrhoea. In those with a sensitive digestive system, start with a low dose. Do not apply to broken or ulcerated skin. Not suitable for children.

COMBINATIONS
+ With hawthorn, to support arterial and venous health
+ With marigold and/or plantain, to promote tissue healing, especially where linked to varicose veins, and in varicose eczema

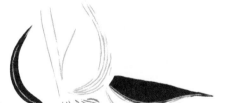

Garlic

Allium sativum

A natural antibiotic, garlic is useful in treating feverish digestive and respiratory infections. Since garlic supports a healthy gut bacterial population, it may be taken alongside prescribed antibiotics to protect against symptoms such as diarrhoea and thrush. Valuable in high blood pressure, varicose veins, and arteriosclerosis, garlic helps normalize cardiovascular function and has longstanding traditional use as an anti-ageing and anti-cancer remedy. Fungal skin infections, such as athlete's foot and warts respond well to garlic applied topically.

PARTS USED
Bulb

MAIN USES
Chest infections, earache, sore throat, fever, infections of all kinds, high blood pressure, arteriosclerosis; to support healthy gut flora

MAIN ACTIONS
Antibiotic, antiviral, diaphoretic, expectorant, lowers blood pressure, lowers raised blood cholesterol and blood sugar levels, thins blood

BEST TAKEN AS
Internal use
+ Concentrated extracts, crushed fresh clove
External use
+ Infused oil

DOSAGE
Internal use
+ 1–3 cloves a day, in food or drink
External use
+ Infused oil (See p. 236 to prepare infused garlic oil for earache)

LENGTH OF TREATMENT
Long-term treatment is fine.

CAUTIONS
Garlic is not considered suitable as a medicine for children under twelve. Seek professional advice if taking anti-coagulant medication.

COMBINATIONS
+ With artichoke and milk thistle for raised blood cholesterol and blood sugar levels
+ With elderflower and propolis for earache and infection

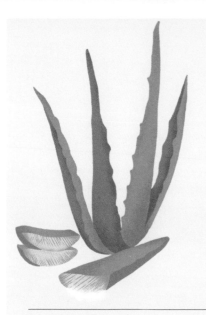

Aloe vera

Aloe vera

Known as the "first-aid" plant, spiky aloe vera merits a place in every home, whether grown on a windowsill, in a greenhouse, or the garden. Extracted directly from the leaf (see p. 243), the clear gel can be applied directly to cleanse and heal cuts, wounds, abrasions, burns, and inflamed skin of any kind. Aloe gel can be taken internally to improve the microbiome, gut health, and to relieve constipation. It is a useful remedy in chronic inflammatory bowel disease, and by promoting tissue healing within the gut, may help with leaky gut syndrome.

PARTS USED
Leaf, gel

MAIN USES
Tissue repair throughout the body, cuts, grazes, burns, acne, eczema, psoriasis, irritable bowel symptoms, constipation, inflammatory gut problems

MAIN ACTIONS
Tissue healer, anti-inflammatory, immune modulator, laxative

BEST TAKEN AS
Internal use
+ Juice, gel, concentrated extracts
External use
+ Juice, gel as lotion, cream

DOSAGE
Internal use
+ Juice, gel up to 25 ml (1 ½ tbsp) a day
External use
+ Juice, gel as required

LENGTH OF TREATMENT
Long-term treatment at low a dose is fine.

CAUTIONS
Consume only the clear gel within the leaf. Do not consume the yellow sap; this is a strong laxative and causes diarrhoea and bowel irritation.

COMBINATIONS
+ With marigold for inflammatory skin conditions (topical use)
+ With chamomile for irritable bowel syndrome and chronic inflammatory bowel disorders

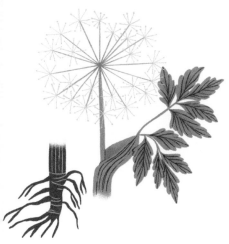

Angelica

Angelica archangelica

A nourishing, gently bitter herb, angelica stimulates appetite and digestive secretions and improves nutrient uptake. It also has a markedly warming and relaxant activity, making it particularly suitable for those who lack vitality and are prone to holding tension in their body. It acts to open up the micro-circulation, encouraging normal healthy function in areas deprived of effective local blood flow, whether in the chest, abdomen, or hands and feet. Poor peripheral circulation can be improved or reversed with long-term low-dose treatment.

PARTS USED
Root

MAIN USES
Poor appetite, anorexia, weak digestion, indigestion and wind, headache and migraine, chest infections (including chronic bronchitis), poor circulation to hands and feet, chilblains, cystitis, chronic fatigue

MAIN ACTIONS
Warming tonic, digestive stimulant, circulatory stimulant, diaphoretic, relaxant

BEST TAKEN AS
Internal use
+ Tincture, decoction, capsules, concentrated extracts

DOSAGE
Internal use
+ Tincture 1–7 ml (up to 1½ tsp) a day
+ Dried root as a decoction, up to 5 g (2½ tsp) a day
+ To aid digestion and strengthen appetite, take 10–20 drops tincture in water (or under the tongue) before meals

LENGTH OF TREATMENT
Low doses can be taken long-term; large doses for up to three weeks.

CAUTIONS
Angelica is safe herb at the correct dosage. Do not take during pregnancy or if you are taking prescribed anti-coagulants.

COMBINATIONS
+ With thyme and garlic for chest infections and bronchial asthma
+ With liquorice and/or ashwagandha for poor appetite and chronic fatigue

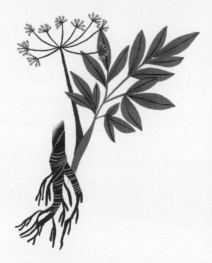

Chinese angelica

Angelica sinensis

Chinese angelica, or *dang gui*, is a warming, nourishing herb that improves blood flow to cold and congested areas and is often helpful in resolving menstrual problems, including pre-menstrual syndrome, irregular menstruation, and cramping pains. Though not directly hormonal, it supports the effectiveness of hormonally active herbs such as chaste tree. Most easily taken as a tincture, this herb's tonic activity extends to the liver, digestion, and heart, in each case supporting healthy function rather than being a treatment for active illness.

PARTS USED
Root

MAIN USES
Irregular menstruation, menstrual cramps, difficulty in conceiving, anaemia, circulatory problems (including poor peripheral circulation and arteriosclerosis), weak digestion with wind and bloating; as a menopausal tonic

MAIN ACTIONS
Warming circulatory tonic, antispasmodic, stimulates menstrual flow, aids iron absorption, liver protective, digestive tonic

BEST TAKEN AS
Internal use
+ Tincture, decoction, powder, concentrated extracts

DOSAGE
Internal use
+ Tincture 2.5 ml (½ tsp) up to four times a day
+ Decoction up to 10 g (⅓ oz) dried herb in 300 ml (10½ fl oz) water a day
+ Powder 1–5 g (up to 1 tsp) a day

LENGTH OF TREATMENT
Long-term treatment at a low dose is fine.

CAUTIONS
Do not take Chinese angelica during pregnancy or while breastfeeding. Avoid taking in heavy menstrual bleeding. This herb may interact with blood-thinning medication.

COMBINATIONS
+ With shatavari for vaginal dryness and reduced libido
+ With chaste berry to improve menstrual regularity and to aid fertility and conception

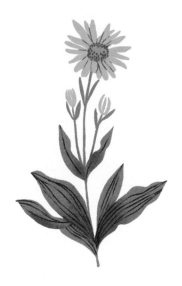

Arnica

Arnica montana

A vivid yellow Alpine flower, arnica promotes tissue healing and repair. Commonly available as a cream or ointment in pharmacies across Europe, arnica speeds the repair of bruised and aching skin and underlying damaged tissue. It achieves this in part by stimulating greater local blood flow. Its pain-relieving properties make it helpful in easing nerve and muscle pains, for example, after strenuous exercise. It is an excellent first-aid remedy, and fits well in a herbal first-aid kit.

PARTS USED
Flower

MAIN USES
Bruises and sprains, muscle aches and pain, nerve pain, painful varicose veins

MAIN ACTIONS
Anti-inflammatory, relieves pain, stimulates tissue repair

BEST TAKEN AS
External use
+ Tincture, lotion, cream, ointment

DOSAGE
External use
+ Tincture 5–10 ml (1–2 tsp) to 50 ml (3 tbsp) water applied as a compress to the affected area
+ Lotion, cream, or ointment two to four times a day, as wanted

LENGTH OF TREATMENT
Can be used long-term but discontinue if you developed signs of a skin reaction.

CAUTIONS
Arnica is a potentially toxic herb. Do not take it internally or apply it to broken skin. The herb may cause allergic skin reactions.

COMBINATIONS
+ With lavender essential oil to aid tissue healing and for pain relief
+ With marigold for cuts, abrasions, and wounds and to promote tissue repair

Barberry

Berberis vulgaris

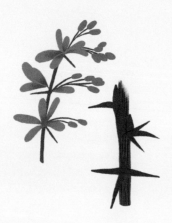

Strongly bitter and strong-acting, barberry needs to be used with care (if you are new to it, try a small amount first). A valuable remedy for indigestion and gastritis, as well as digestive and parasitic infections, such as food poisoning and giardia, barberry finds use in many types of infection, whether acute or chronic. It is especially effective when combined with appropriate herbs, such as *cloves*, echinacea, or elderberry. Its antibacterial and anti-inflammatory activities make it useful in treating acne and boils.

PARTS USED
Bark, fruit

MAIN USES
Indigestion, gall bladder problems, bacterial, fungal, and viral infections, gastrointestinal infections, metabolic syndrome, acne, as a broad-ranging antimicrobial

MAIN ACTIONS
Antimicrobial, antiparasitic, anti-inflammatory, reduces fever, bitter tonic, stimulates bile flow

BEST TAKEN AS
Internal use
+ Tincture, powdered root, dried berries

DOSAGE
Internal use
+ Tincture 3–5 ml (½–1 tsp) a day
+ Powdered root or berries 2–5 g (½–1 tsp) a day in small doses

LENGTH OF TREATMENT
One month at high dose; up to three months at a low dose.

CAUTIONS
Do not take barberry during pregnancy or while breastfeeding. This herb is not suitable for children.

COMBINATIONS
+ With echinacea and/or olive leaf for bacterial and viral infection, especially of the gastrointestinal tract
+ With marigold and chaste berry for acne

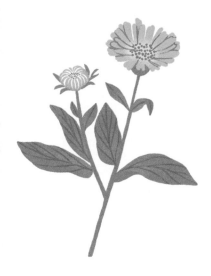

Marigold

Calendula officinalis

Marigold's warming, soothing, and cleansing flowers are used to heal all manner of minor wounds, burns, and inflamed tissue. Marigold is also a go-to treatment for fungal problems including athlete's foot and thrush. Applied as a lotion, an infusion will cleanse damaged tissue, while promoting tissue repair. Taken internally marigold is a key remedy for repair of mucous membranes within the stomach and throughout the digestive tract. Mildly antispasmodic, it soothes menstrual cramps and reduces heavy menstrual blood flow.

PARTS USED
Flower, petal

MAIN USES
Inflammatory skin conditions (including acne, thrush, nappy rash, cradle cap, sore nipples), digestive problems, toxic states, menstrual cramps and heavy bleeding; as a first-aid treatment for cuts, grazes, and wounds

MAIN ACTIONS
Anti-inflammatory, wound healer, slows bleeding, antibacterial, antifungal, mild oestrogenic, detoxifying

BEST TAKEN AS
Internal use
+ Infusion, tincture
External use
+ Lotion, cream, ointment

DOSAGE
Internal use
+ Infusion 10 g (⅓ oz) dried flowers to 200 ml (7 fl oz) water a day
+ Tincture 2.5 ml (½ tsp) once or twice a day
External use
+ Lotion, cream, or ointment two to four times a day, as wanted

LENGTH OF TREATMENT
Can be safely used long-term.

CAUTIONS
Marigold can cause an allergic reaction, although this is rare.

COMBINATIONS
+ With chamomile and meadowsweet for acid indigestion and all inflammatory gut problems
+ With echinacea and olive leaf for thrush and fungal infections

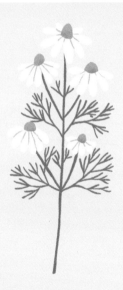

Chamomile

Chamomilla recutita

An exceptionally useful and safe remedy known as the "mother of the gut", chamomile calms, soothes, and gently warms, making it particularly helpful in common childhood complaints such as colic, teething, diarrhoea, and disturbed sleep. In adults, chamomile brings relief to digestive problems of all kinds, its anti-inflammatory and antispasmodic effects reducing nerve irritability and healing inflamed tissue. Chamomile is a valuable remedy in allergic conditions such as hay fever, and makes an excellent salve for sore and inflamed skin.

PARTS USED
Flower

MAIN USES
All manner of problems affecting the digestive tract (especially in children), anxiety and tension, poor sleep, mild allergies (including hay fever), tight chest, inflammatory skin disorders; topically, to heal wounds, burns, and inflamed skin

MAIN ACTIONS
Anti-inflammatory, tissue healer, relaxant, antispasmodic, relieves pain, antimicrobial, soothes digestive tract

BEST TAKEN AS
Internal use
+ Infusion, tincture
External use
+ Lotion, cream

DOSAGE
Internal use
+ Infusion 1–2 teabags to a cup or 10 g (⅓ oz) dried flowers in 200 ml (7 fl oz) water a day
+ Tincture 5 ml (1 tsp) one to three times a day
External use
+ Lotion or cream two to three times a day, as wanted

LENGTH OF TREATMENT
Long-term treatment at a low dose is fine.

CAUTIONS
Chamomile is a safe herb and rarely causes allergic reactions. Do not take chamomile essential oil internally.

COMBINATIONS
+ With fennel seed and/or ginger root for indigestion, wind, bloating, digestive cramps, nausea, and travel sickness
+ With echinacea and elderflower for sinus infection, sinus headache, hay fever, upper respiratory catarrh and earache

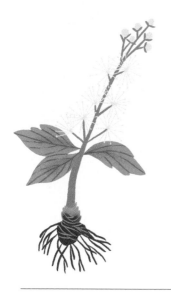

Black cohosh

Actaea racemosa

A valued remedy for menopausal problems, black cohosh can sometimes halt symptoms such as hot flushing, night sweats, and disturbed sleep within a matter of days. The root supports oestrogenic activity within the body, though it does not contain oestrogenic compounds – rather it is thought to modulate oestrogen receptors increasing their activity in low oestrogen states. Other uses, related in part to its sedative and relaxant effects, are tinnitus, migraine, and nerve pain. It is also a herb to consider in muscular and arthritic cramps.

PARTS USED
Root

MAIN USES
Menopausal symptoms, menstrual cramps, pre-menstrual symptoms, arthritis, muscle pains and cramps, neuralgia, tinnitus

MAIN ACTIONS
Oestrogenic, uterine tonic, anti-inflammatory, mild relaxant/sedative, antirheumatic

BEST TAKEN AS
Internal use
+ Tincture, concentrated extracts

DOSAGE
Internal use
+ Tincture 1–3 ml (¼–½ tsp) a day

LENGTH OF TREATMENT
Long-term treatment at a lower dose is fine.

CAUTIONS
Do not take black cohosh during pregnancy or if you are breastfeeding. Large doses can cause stomach upsets and headaches.

COMBINATIONS
+ With St Johns wort for menopausal symptoms including disturbed sleep, lowered mood, and exhaustion
+ With Chinese angelica for menstrual cramps and pre-menstrual symptoms

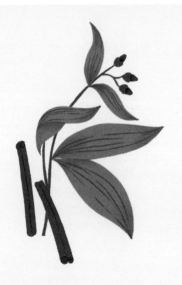

Cinnamon

Cinnamomum verum

Cinnamon finds use in many self-help situations and could be described as a "cure-all". As a warming tonic herb, it makes an excellent hot infusion in colds, flu, chills, and poor peripheral circulation. Helpful in nausea, travel sickness, wind, and bloating, as well as acute and chronic diarrhoea, cinnamon's anti-inflammatory and astringent activity tones and soothes the entire digestive tract. The herb has an ability to lower blood glucose levels and recent research suggests it also has neuroprotective activity.

PARTS USED
Inner bark

MAIN USES
Nausea and vomiting, flatulence and bloating, diarrhoea, colds and flu, rheumatic aches and pains, high blood pressure, pre-menstrual syndrome, oral thrush

MAIN ACTIONS
Warming tonic, antimicrobial, astringent, relieves wind and bloating, antirheumatic, antidiabetic, neuroprotective

BEST TAKEN AS
Internal use
+ Tincture, powder, concentrated extracts

DOSAGE
Internal use
+ Tincture 2.5–5 ml (½–1 tsp) a day
+ Powder up to 2.5 g (½ tsp) a day

LENGTH OF TREATMENT
Long-term treatment at a low dose is fine.

CAUTIONS
Cinnamon rarely causes allergic reactions. Do not take essential oil internally.

COMBINATIONS
+ With echinacea and elderberry for colds, flu, and viral infections
+ With artichoke leaf to support stable blood sugar levels

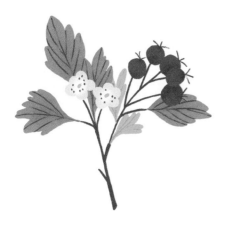

Hawthorn

Crataegus oxyacantha, C. monogyna

Commonly thought of as a "food" for the heart and circulation, hawthorn's value in treating high blood pressure and early-stage heart failure is well-established, and it is the herbal remedy to consider in cardiovascular ill health. Both leaf and berry help the heart to work with greater regularity and efficiency and reduce fatty deposits and inflammation affecting the inner lining of the arteries. Hawthorn also has longstanding use as a remedy for chronic digestive problems, particularly where poor circulation may be a factor.

PARTS USED
Flower, leaf, berry

MAIN USES
High blood pressure, low blood pressure, angina, weak heart function, palpitations

MAIN ACTIONS
Heart and circulatory tonic, acts to normalize blood pressure, relaxant

BEST TAKEN AS
Internal use
+ Infusion, tincture, powder, concentrated extracts

DOSAGE
Internal use
+ Infusion up to 5 g (2½ tsp) fresh berry or leaf in 200 ml (7 fl oz) a day
+ Tincture (berry or leaf) 2.5 ml (½ tsp) up to four times a day
+ Powdered berry or leaf up to 2.5 g (½ tsp) a day

LENGTH OF TREATMENT
Long-term treatment at a low dose is fine.

CAUTIONS
If you are taking prescribed medication for cardiovascular problems, seek professional advice before taking hawthorn.

COMBINATIONS
+ With cinnamon and olive leaf for high blood pressure
+ With lemon balm to support heart regularity and for palpitations

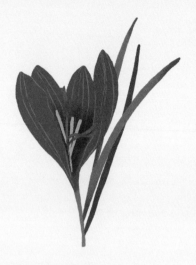

Saffron

Crocus sativus

Saffron has a wide-ranging ability to heal and enliven. It supports and strengthens cognitive function, can be taken to aid memory and concentration and as a neuroprotective agent, and it has antidepressant activity. Saffron strengthens eyesight; in some, it will improve colour perception and depth of vision, promoting retinal acuity and protecting against age-related macular degeneration. Saffron has longstanding use as a tonic remedy for the heart, helping where emotional distress affects and weakens normal heart function.

PARTS USED
Stigma, filament

MAIN USES
Lowered mood and depression, eye conditions such as macular degeneration, "emotional" heart problems, to protect against dementia, to support and strengthen the central nervous system and mental function, as a sexual tonic

MAIN ACTIONS
Neuroprotective, promotes memory and concentration, supports vision, antidepressant, heart tonic, anti-inflammatory

BEST TAKEN AS
Internal use
+ Filaments

DOSAGE
Internal use
+ 5–10 filaments twice a day

LENGTH OF TREATMENT
Best taken long-term.

CAUTIONS
Do not take saffron as a medicine during pregnancy. Do not exceed recommended dosage, as large doses can be toxic.

COMBINATIONS
+ With lemon balm and/or rosemary to support and enhance memory and concentration and maintain healthy cognition
+ With hawthorn berry for broken-heart syndrome and emotional heart health

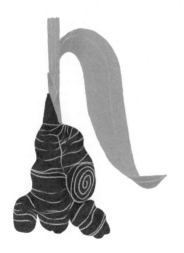

Turmeric

Curcuma longa

A close relative of ginger, turmeric can prove useful in all inflammatory conditions, including chronic inflammatory diseases. Though traditionally seen as a medicine for liver, gall bladder, and digestive disorders, turmeric is now often taken as an anti-inflammatory to help treat conditions as varied as type 2 diabetes, osteoarthritis, Alzheimer's disease, psoriasis, and cancer. Long-term use of conventional anti-inflammatories can sometimes lead to significant side-effects – a key benefit of this root is that it may be taken long-term with minimal risk of side-effects.

PARTS USED
Root

MAIN USES
Arthritis, muscle pain and inflammation, backache, headache, sore mouth, mouth ulcers, gastrointestinal and liver disorders, fungal and candida infections; externally, for inflammatory and fungal skin conditions

MAIN ACTIONS
Anti-inflammatory, lowers raised cholesterol levels, antibacterial and antifungal, anticancer

BEST TAKEN AS
Internal use
+ Powder or capsule formulated with black pepper or piperine
External use
+ Cream, ointment

DOSAGE
Internal use
+ Powder up to 5 g (1 tsp) a day
External use
+ Cream, ointment, as wanted

LENGTH OF TREATMENT
Long-term treatment (minimum of four weeks) is recommended for chronic inflammatory conditions.

CAUTIONS
If taking anticoagulant medication, or if gallstones are present, take turmeric only on professional advice. Turmeric occasionally causes skin rashes.

COMBINATIONS
+ With ginger and/or liquorice for chronic inflammatory disease, including arthritic pain and inflammation
+ With artichoke and/or olive leaf for raised cholesterol levels and liver disorders

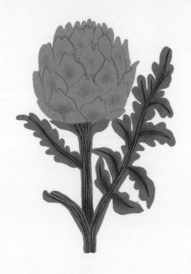

Artichoke

Cynara scolymus

Better known for its edible flowerheads than its leaves, artichoke has a powerful protective action on the liver, pancreas, and digestive system, supporting liver health and aiding in a wide range of liver disorders. Strongly bitter, the leaves stimulate digestive secretions and bile flow and relieve wind and bloating. The leaf helps to lower raised cholesterol levels – partly by reducing cholesterol production in the liver, and is a good food and medicine for diabetics. It is a key herb to take long-term in aiding weight loss.

PARTS USED
Leaf

MAIN USES
Fatty liver disease and abnormal liver function, high cholesterol levels, pre-diabetic states, weight loss, metabolic syndrome, nausea, weak digestion with flatulence and bloating

MAIN ACTIONS
Bitter and digestive tonic, protects and supports liver function, lowers raised blood cholesterol and blood sugar levels, diuretic

BEST TAKEN AS
Internal use
+ Infusion, powder, concentrated extracts
+ The flowerheads eaten as a vegetable also make good medicine

DOSAGE
Internal use
+ Infusion 5–10 g (2½–5 tsp) dried herb in 200 ml (7 fl oz) water a day as a digestive aid and for flatulence and bloating
+ Powder 2–5 g (½–1 tsp) a day

LENGTH OF TREATMENT
Long-term treatment is fine.

CAUTIONS
Consult your healthcare practitioner before taking artichoke leaf as a medicine if you have gallstones.

COMBINATIONS
+ With olive leaf and rosemary to aid weight loss
+ With milk thistle or dandelion root for raised cholesterol levels and liver disease

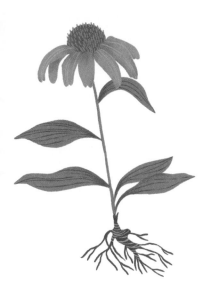

Echinacea

Echinacea purpurea, E. angustifolia, E. pallida

Echinacea supports and strengthens immune function, thus helping the body to counter the challenge of infection or toxicity more effectively. It is particularly useful in acute viral and bacterial infections such as sinusitis and tonsillitis but can prove a valuable addition in treating a wide range of health problems, including inflammatory skin conditions such as acne and eczema, fungal infections such as thrush and athlete's foot, and chronic health problems including chronic fatigue and nervous exhaustion.

PARTS USED
Root, leaf

MAIN USES
Bacterial and viral infections (especially upper and lower respiratory infection), fungal infection, chronic infections, depressed immune function, poisoning/toxicity, dry mouth

MAIN ACTIONS
Immune tonic, anti-inflammatory, antimicrobial, detoxifier, stimulates saliva, wound healer

BEST TAKEN AS
Internal use
+ Decoction, tincture, concentrated extracts
External use
+ Cream, lotion

DOSAGE
Internal use
+ Decoction 5–10 g (2½–5 tsp) dried herb to 300 ml water a day
+ Tincture 2.5 ml (½ tsp) one to four times a day
+ Tincture 5 ml (1 tsp) to 75 ml (3 fl oz) water as a mouthwash or gargle
External use
+ Cream or lotion to prevent or treat infection

LENGTH OF TREATMENT
Long-term treatment at a low dose is fine.

CAUTIONS
Echinacea can cause allergic reactions, although this is rare.

COMBINATIONS
+ With ashwagandha, marigold, and liquorice for chronic or "stuck" infections
+ With elecampane, garlic, and thyme for respiratory infections

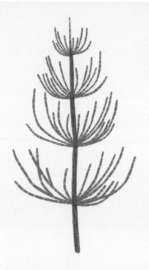

Horsetail

Equisetum arvense

Horsetail is a key remedy for the bladder and urinary tract, its high silica content helping to maintain a smooth, water-resistant surface to the inner lining of the bladder and urinary tubules, soothing irritation and making it more difficult for bacteria to adhere to the urinary tract walls. Though only mildly antiseptic, horsetail combines well with herbs such *cornsilk* for acute and chronic urinary tract infections. The herb is undervalued as a preventative or treatment for osteopenia and osteoporosis – take with black cohosh.

PARTS USED
Aerial parts

MAIN USES
Urinary tract infections, lower urinary tract symptoms (including day- or night-time frequency and poor urine flow), osteoporosis, as a source of soluble silica and calcium for repair of connective tissue (joint, bone, and lung)

MAIN ACTIONS
Urinary astringent, stops bleeding, bladder tonic

BEST TAKEN AS
Internal use
+ Decoction, tincture, powder, concentrated extracts

DOSAGE
Internal use
+ Decoction 5–10 g (2½–5 tsp) dried herb to 300 ml (10½ fl oz) water a day
+ Tincture 2.5 ml (½ tsp) up to four times a day
+ Powder 1–5 g (¼–1 tsp) a day

LENGTH OF TREATMENT
Long-term treatment at a low dose is fine.

CAUTIONS
During long-term use, take a thiamine/vitamin B complex supplement.

COMBINATIONS
+ With saw palmetto for urethritis, prostatitis, enlarged prostate, and poor urine flow
+ With fennel seed and buchu for chronic cystitis and bladder complaints

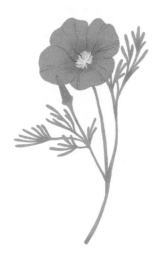

Californian poppy

Eschscholzia californica

Californian poppy is a safe remedy, particularly for children, being taken to soothe and calm at times of anxiety, irritability, and difficulty in getting off to sleep. It is a herb to try to relieve nightmares. In adults, it finds similar use easing head and neck ache, anxiety, tension, and spasmodic (muscle) pain. Californian poppy is one of the few herbs that may be helpful in treating neuralgia and neuropathic pain – large doses may be required, but the herb does not usually cause drowsiness or excessive sedation.

PARTS USED
Aerial parts

MAIN USES
Sleep disturbance (including nightmares), anxiety, headache, for pain relief

MAIN ACTIONS
Mild analgesic, mild sedative, relaxant

BEST TAKEN AS
Internal use
+ Infusion, tincture

DOSAGE
Internal use
+ Best as small, frequent doses. Infusion 10 g (⅓ oz) dried herb to 200 ml (7 fl oz) water a day
+ Tincture 2.5 ml (½ tsp) up to six times a day (up to 10 times a day for neuralgia)

LENGTH OF TREATMENT
As required

CAUTIONS
Californian poppy is a safe herb, and is suitable for children. Excess doses may cause drowsiness.

COMBINATIONS
+ With passion flower for anxiety and insomnia
+ With saffron for pain relief (muscle pain, but potentially neuropathic pain too)

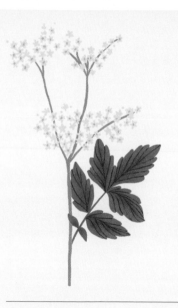

Meadowsweet

Filipendula ulmaria

Meadowsweet is gentle yet effective in easing stomach and lower digestive complaints – in both adults and children. With astringent, anti-inflammatory and antiulcer properties, it helps protect the stomach and lower oesophagus from damage caused by stomach acid. Notably, it does not suppress stomach acid production, but improves the capacity of mucous membranes to resist acid erosion. Within the intestines, meadowsweet reduces irritability and inflammation within the gut wall and can be a useful aid in irritable bowel syndrome.

PARTS USED
Flowering top

MAIN USES
Acid indigestion/reflux, acidic states, intestinal "hurry" and irritable bowel, osteoarthritis, muscle aches and pains, headache, fever

MAIN ACTIONS
Anti-inflammatory, stomachic, antacid, astringent, controls fever

BEST TAKEN AS
Internal use
+ Infusion, tincture, powder

DOSAGE
Internal use
+ Infusion 10–15 g (⅓–½ oz) dried herb to 500 ml (17½ fl oz) water, taken as three divided doses
+ Tincture up to 10 ml (2 tsp) a day in two to four doses. Best taken between meals.

LENGTH OF TREATMENT
Long-term treatment is fine.

CAUTIONS
Do not take meadowsweet if you are allergic to aspirin.

COMBINATIONS
+ With marigold and plantain for acid indigestion and reflux; to aid healing and repair of the stomach
+ With peppermint and lemon balm for irritable bowel symptoms

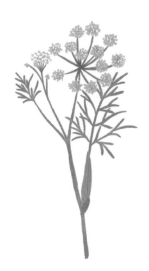

Fennel

Foeniculum vulgare

A remedy for digestive symptoms such as stomach ache, cramps, and bloating, fennel seeds exert a soothing, relaxant activity and gently promote appetite. Safe for children at low dose, an infusion can be taken to relieve colic, sore throat, croup, and chesty conditions. The infusion makes a good eyewash and treatment for sore eyes and conjunctivitis. With oestrogenic activity, fennel seeds are valuable during the perimenopause and menopause, easing hot flushing and associated symptoms. Fennel seeds can also be chewed to support oral health.

PARTS USED
Seed, root

MAIN USES
Digestive discomfort including nausea, wind, and bloating, coughs and chesty conditions, perimenopausal and menopausal symptoms, to increase breast milk flow, as an eye wash

MAIN ACTIONS
Soothes digestion, antispasmodic, expectorant, oestrogenic, stimulates breast milk, diuretic, antifungal

BEST TAKEN AS
Internal use
+ Infusion, tincture, ground seed or powder, concentrated extracts, root as a vegetable

External use
+ Infusion

DOSAGE
Internal use
+ Infusion 4 g (1 tsp) per 200ml (7 fl oz) water a day or 2 to 3 teabags a day
+ Tincture 2.5–5 ml (½–1 tsp) a day
+ Ground seed or powder up to 2 g (½ tsp) a day

External use
+ An infusion made using a teabag makes a good eyewash and treatment for sore eyes and conjunctivitis

LENGTH OF TREATMENT
Long-term treatment at a low dose is fine.

CAUTIONS
Fennel can cause allergic reactions, though this is rare. Do not take fennel essential oil internally.

COMBINATIONS
+ With chamomile and ginger for nausea, wind, bloating, and digestive cramps
+ With sage for menopausal symptoms including hot flushing

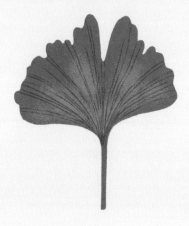

Ginkgo

Ginkgo biloba

Ginkgo leaf has been intensively researched since the 1980s. Extracts are known to exert a stabilizing effect on the central nervous system, reducing inflammatory damage and improving circulation to, and within, the brain. Taken long-term to maintain a healthy circulation, slow ageing processes, and prevent the onset of dementia, ginkgo has a wide range of potential uses, including cold extremities and chilblains, dizziness and tinnitus, and as a restorative remedy to take after a stroke (discuss this with your healthcare practitioner).

PARTS USED
Leaf

MAIN USES
Poor peripheral circulation, dizziness and tinnitus, mild depression, cardiovascular disease, to support memory and mental function

MAIN ACTIONS
Circulatory stimulant, neuroprotective, improves mental performance, anti-inflammatory

BEST TAKEN AS
Internal use
+ Concentrated extracts

DOSAGE
Internal use
+ Extracts standardized to 6 per cent terpenoids and 24 per cent flavonoid glycosides

LENGTH OF TREATMENT
As required; long-term treatment to support healthy mental function.

CAUTIONS
If taking prescribed medication, especially anticoagulants, take gingko only on the recommendation of your healthcare practitioner. Rarely, gingko can cause a headache or gastrointestinal upset.

COMBINATIONS
+ With lemon balm for neuroprotection and poor memory
+ With black cohosh for dizziness and tinnitus

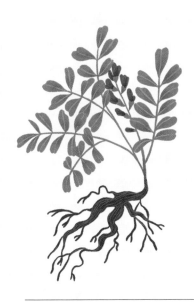

Liquorice

Glycyrrhiza glabra

With an almost dizzying range of health benefits, it is no surprise that in traditional Chinese medicine liquorice is seen as a key "guide drug" enhancing the effectiveness of other ingredients and reducing potential toxicity. Liquorice helps to heal ulcers, protects the liver from inflammatory damage, supports stress hormone release from the adrenal glands, soothes coughs, helps chest problems, and stimulates hair growth. An oestrogenic remedy, liquorice is valuable during the menopause.

PARTS USED
Root

MAIN USES
Acid indigestion, mouth and peptic ulcers, bronchitis, menopausal symptoms, chronic stress and fatigue, constipation, inflammatory conditions (especially of the digestive and respiratory systems)

MAIN ACTIONS
Anti-inflammatory, expectorant, demulcent, adrenal tonic, oestrogenic, mild laxative

BEST TAKEN AS
Internal use
+ Tincture, powder, pure liquorice sweets

DOSAGE
Internal use
+ Tincture 4 ml (80 drops) a day; 1–2 ml (20–40 drops) longer term
+ Powder (or sweets) 2.5 g (½ tsp) a day for a maximum of two weeks; 1–2 g (¼–½ tsp) powder a day (or sweets) longer term.

LENGTH OF TREATMENT
Up to three months for chronic conditions

CAUTIONS
Liquorice is best used at low dosage. Excessive doses cause serious side-effects, including high blood pressure. Do not take in high blood pressure. Do not take during pregnancy. Take long-term only on professional advice.

COMBINATIONS
+ With chamomile and meadowsweet for acid reflux and gastritis
+ With thyme and angelica for bronchitis

Witch hazel

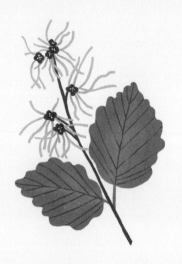

Hamamelis virginiana

Witch hazel is a valuable remedy for inflamed and tender skin conditions. Strongly astringent, distilled witch hazel water tones up and tightens the skin, helping to seal wounds and burns, prevent infection taking hold, and promote tissue repair. This tightening effect makes it useful in overly lax skin problems including blemishes, and creased or sagging skin, as well as underlying problems such as raised capillaries, haemorrhoids, and varicose veins. The distilled water is an excellent eyewash for tired, bruised, and inflamed eyes, and for conjunctivitis.

PARTS USED
Leaf, twig

MAIN USES
Inflamed and over-relaxed skin, bruises and spontaneous bruising, sprains and hernias, raised capillaries, varicose veins, haemorrhoids, sore eyes, conjunctivitis, nose bleeds

MAIN ACTIONS
Astringent, anti-inflammatory, staunches bleeding

BEST TAKEN AS
External use
+ Distilled water, lotion, cream

DOSAGE
External use
+ Distilled water, lotion, cream, as wanted

LENGTH OF TREATMENT
Daily topical use is fine.

CAUTIONS
Take witch hazel internally only on professional advice. Do not apply to wounds or burns where the surface of the skin has been removed.

COMBINATIONS
+ With rose distilled water (equal parts) as a skin tonic
+ With echinacea as a lotion for weeping skin infections

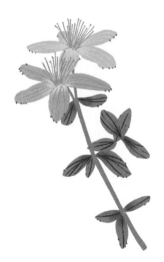

St John's wort

Hypericum perforatum

St John's wort is a key herb for mild to moderate depression, anxiety states, and disturbed sleep. It supports a positive outlook and healthy cognitive function during periods of nervous exhaustion, long-term stress, and pre-menstrual tension, as well as at the menopause. In such situations, the herb wraps a "protective cloak" around you, enabling you to cope more readily. Taken internally and applied topically as an infused oil, St John's wort can prove helpful in soothing neuralgia caused by shingles, sciatica, or other conditions involving nerve damage.

PARTS USED
Flowering tops

MAIN USES
Low mood and mild to moderate depression, anxiety and irritability, nerve pain (including sciatica), perimenopausal and menopausal symptoms, insomnia, cold sores, shingles, to support nerve repair

MAIN ACTIONS
Antidepressant, neuroprotective, anti-inflammatory, antiviral, wound healer, aids sleep

BEST TAKEN AS
Internal use
+ Tincture, concentrated extracts
External use
+ Infused oil

DOSAGE
Internal use
+ Tincture 2.5 ml (½ tsp) one to three times a day
+ Concentrated extract

External use
+ Infused oil applied neat or with added essential oils (see p. 236)

LENGTH OF TREATMENT
Long-term treatment is fine.

CAUTIONS
St John's wort is a safe herb on its own but if taking prescribed medication, seek advice from your healthcare practitioner before taking it. Extracts, especially standardized tablets, can interact with prescribed medicines, including some antibiotics and the contraceptive pill.

COMBINATIONS
+ With cramp bark and Californian poppy for nerve pain, including sciatica
+ With ashwagandha for anxiety, irritability, and nervous exhaustion

Elecampane

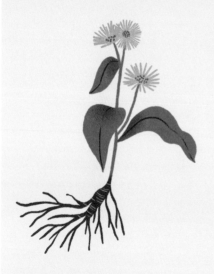

Inula helenium

A gently bitter, tonic remedy, elecampane has an affinity for the chest, disinfecting the airways and aiding recovery from infection lodged in the bronchial tubes and lungs. Useful for acute and chronic bronchitis, it also proves helpful in treating upper respiratory infections. A restorative herb, elecampane makes an excellent warming tonic in convalescence and for older adults recovering from severe ill health, especially where the chest and lungs have been weakened. It has longstanding use as a safe remedy in treating intestinal worms.

PARTS USED
Root

MAIN USES
Acute and chronic chest problems (including bronchitis), wheeziness, cough, indigestion, convalescence, digestive weakness, intestinal worms

MAIN ACTIONS
Cough soother, chest remedy, digestive tonic, stimulates sweating, antibacterial, antiviral, expels worms

BEST TAKEN AS
Internal use
+ Decoction, tincture, powder, concentrated extracts

DOSAGE
Internal use
+ Decoction 10 g (⅓ oz) root to 300 ml (10½ fl oz) water a day
+ Tincture 3–10 ml (½–2 tsp) a day
+ Powdered root 3–8 g (½–1½ tsp) a day

LENGTH OF TREATMENT
Long-term treatment at a low dose is fine.

CAUTIONS
Do not take elecampane during pregnancy or while breastfeeding. It can cause allergic reactions, but this is rare.

COMBINATIONS
+ With liquorice and thyme for chest problems and respiratory catarrh
+ With garlic and thyme for intestinal worms, especially threadworms

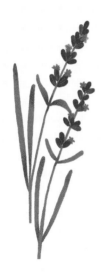

Lavender

Lavandula officinalis

Best known for its soothing essential oil, lavender calms, relaxes, and lifts the mood, enabling a clearer perspective. It is a first-rate remedy for shock and sudden distress, as well as restless and irritable states, where there may be a sense of being out of control. Lavender has significant analgesic activity and brings relief to aches and pains, notably headache and joint and muscle pain. It is also a key sleep-aid remedy, especially where pain or discomfort is a factor. The essential oil makes an invaluable first-aid remedy for small cuts, burns, sunburn, insect bites and stings, and so on.

PARTS USED
Flower

MAIN USES
Internal use
Anxiety, worry and angst, low mood, headache, wind and bloating
External use
Muscle aches, pain (including headache and toothache), and small burns; to promote tissue healing, as an insect repellent, and to soothe and heal bites and stings

MAIN ACTIONS
Relaxant, antianxiety, mild antidepressant, analgesic, neuroprotective, tissue healer, antimicrobial

BEST TAKEN AS
Internal use
+ Tincture, concentrated extracts
External use
+ Lotion, cream, essential oil

DOSAGE
Internal use
+ Tincture 2.5 ml (½ tsp) one to three times a day
External use
+ Lotion, cream as needed; essential oil can be massaged neat onto small areas

LENGTH OF TREATMENT
Long-term treatment at a low dose is fine.

CAUTIONS
Do not take lavender essential oil internally.

COMBINATIONS
+ With peppermint and rosemary for nervous anxiety and headache
+ With Californian poppy and Chinese angelica for pain relief and comfort

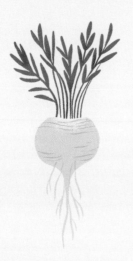

Maca

Lepidium meyenii

Maca is a highly nutritious tonic food, with great restorative potential. Chronic exhaustion, fatigue, and ongoing stress may all benefit from regular intake, as it supports the body's ability to adapt to and cope with stress. It may also strengthen memory and cognitive performance. Research suggests that the root has a directly positive effect on sexual function, enhancing libido and sexual desire, and notably in healthy menopausal women. It is also thought to aid male fertility, erectile dysfunction, and enlarged prostate.

PARTS USED
Root

MAIN USES
To increase libido and treat sexual dysfunction (particularly in older adults), to improve stamina and vitality, may aid memory and cognition, and raise lowered mood

MAIN ACTIONS
Adaptogen, sexual tonic, anabolic (supports muscle tissue and strength)

BEST TAKEN AS
Internal use
+ Powder

DOSAGE
Internal use
+ Powder 2.5–5 g (½–1 tsp) powder a day, best blended in a smoothie or added to food

LENGTH OF TREATMENT
Can be taken long-term.

CAUTIONS
Maca is not associated with any health risks at the recommended dosage.

COMBINATIONS
+ With ashwagandha in chronic fatigue, male infertility, and erectile dysfunction
+ With shatavari to aid libido in women, especially post-menopause

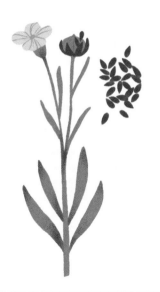

Flaxseed

Linum usitatissimum

High in fibre and essential fatty acids, flaxseed is an excellent remedy for chronic constipation and some cases of irritable bowel syndrome. Its gooey consistency – once soaked in water for twenty to thirty minutes – soothes and protects the digestive tract, slows absorption of nutrients such as fats and sugars, retains fluid within the colon, and encourages a softer and easier-to-pass stool. Flaxseed is also a key source of anti-inflammatory phytoestrogens, making it a valuable supplement at the menopause.

PARTS USED
Seed

MAIN USES
Constipation, dry coughs and bronchitis, menopausal symptoms (including hot flushing and vaginal dryness), as an aid in lowering raised blood cholesterol and glucose levels

MAIN ACTIONS
Demulcent, phytoestrogenic, bulk laxative, expectorant

BEST TAKEN AS ACTIONS
Internal use
+ Cracked or ground seed

DOSAGE
Internal use
+ Seed up to 25 g (1 oz) a day, soaked in at least 125 ml (4 fl oz) water

LENGTH OF TREATMENT
Long-term treatment is recommended.

CAUTIONS
Flaxseeds are best diluted with at least five times their volume of water. Unripe seeds are toxic. Store cracked/ground seed in an airtight container in the fridge – once ground, it oxidizes very quickly.

COMBINATIONS
+ With aloe vera juice in chronic constipation
+ With elecampane for chronic coughs and bronchitis

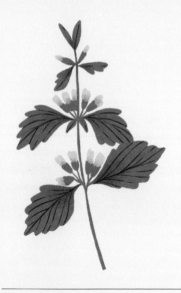

Lemon balm

Melissa officinalis

Lemon balm is traditionally used as a relaxing heart tonic and antiageing remedy. A key remedy where emotional stress affects normal heart function – thus its use in nervous palpitations – it helps to ease anxiety, negativity, and lowered mood. Its neuroprotective activity supports healthy brain function and prevents or slows the onset of dementia. Lemon balm may also help in mild cases of over-active thyroid. The juice squeezed from fresh leaves or a cream can prove effective applied to herpes sores at the first sign of an outbreak.

PARTS USED
Aerial parts

MAIN USES
Anxiety, low mood, restlessness, nervous palpitations, nervous indigestion, cold sores and herpes infection, headache, as a neuroprotective agent

MAIN ACTIONS
Relaxant, tonic, neuroprotective, antispasmodic, antiviral, diaphoretic

BEST TAKEN AS
Internal use
+ Infusion, tincture, concentrated extracts
External use
+ Juice, cream, essential oil

DOSAGE
Internal use
+ Infusion 5 g (2½ tsp) dried herb to 200 ml (7 fl oz) water a day
+ Tincture 2.5 ml (½ tsp) one to three times a day
External use
+ Juice, cream, essential oil – apply to cold sores and shingles. Juice can be squeezed from fresh leaves in a garlic crusher.

LENGTH OF TREATMENT
Long-term treatment at a low dose is fine.

CAUTIONS
Do not take lemon balm essential oil internally.

COMBINATIONS
+ With ginkgo and rosemary to support memory and healthy cognition and to counter neurodegeneration
+ With hawthorn and passion flower for palpitations

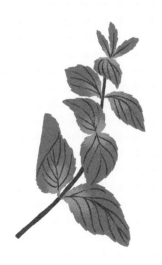

Peppermint

Mentha x piperita

Peppermint's ability to anaesthetize nerve endings and reduce inflammation throughout the digestive tract makes it useful in conditions as varied as burping, stomach cramps, chronic diarrhoea, and irritable bowel. An infusion is effective in these conditions, though peppermint oil capsules are stronger. A remedy for catarrhal problems and upper respiratory infection, the infusion drunk or inhaled helps to soothe and open up the airways. A few drops of essential oil applied to painful joints, the neck, or temples often helps to relieve pain and discomfort.

PARTS USED
Aerial parts

MAIN USES
Internal use
Trapped wind and burping, indigestion, digestive cramps, irritable bowel, colds and flu, feverish states, headache, migraine
External use
Skin sensitivity, itchiness

MAIN ACTIONS
Relieves wind and bloating, tonic, antispasmodic, antiviral, anti-inflammatory, diaphoretic, local anaesthetic

BEST TAKEN AS
Internal use
+ Infusion, tincture, concentrated extracts, capsules
External use
+ Lotion, cream, essential oil

DOSAGE
Internal use
+ Infusion 5 g (2½ tsp) dried herb to 200 ml (7 fl oz) water a day
+ Tincture 2.5 ml (½ tsp) up to four times a day
+ Peppermint oil capsules as indicated
External use
+ Lotion, cream, essential oil, as wanted

LENGTH OF TREATMENT
Long-term treatment is fine.

CAUTIONS
Peppermint is a safe herb, although it can cause heartburn. It is not suitable for children under five years old.

COMBINATIONS
+ With chamomile for indigestion, stomach and intestinal cramps, and irritable bowel
+ With elderflower, garlic, and ginger for colds, flu, and fever.

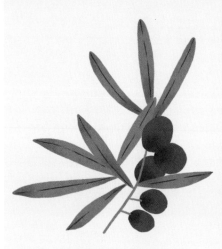

Olive

Olea europea

Profoundly bitter, olive leaf has wide-ranging applications. A potent antioxidant and anti-inflammatory, it supports the health of both the arteries and the heart and has an established ability to lower blood pressure. Its action on the liver and digestive system can help lower raised cholesterol and raised blood sugar levels. Olive oil nourishes the skin and has mild antifungal activity. Though rather greasy, it makes a good local treatment for fungal skin infections, including cradle cap and dandruff, and can be used to remove excess earwax.

PARTS USED
Leaf, fruit

MAIN USES
High blood pressure and atheroma, raised cholesterol levels, bacterial and fungal infections (including candidiasis); as a "protective" remedy supporting heart, liver, and neurological health

MAIN ACTIONS
Anti-inflammatory, antibacterial, antiviral, antifungal, bitter heart and circulatory tonic, lowers raised blood pressure and blood fat levels, anticancer

BEST TAKEN AS
Internal use
+ Infusion, tincture, concentrated extracts

DOSAGE
Internal use
+ Infusion up to 10 g (⅓ oz) dried leaf to 200 ml (7 fl oz) water a day
+ Tincture 2.5 ml (½ tsp) one to four times a day

LENGTH OF TREATMENT
Long-term treatment at a low dose is fine.

CAUTIONS
Olive can cause allergic reactions, although this is rare. Do not take olive essential oil internally.

COMBINATIONS
+ With garlic and hawthorn in high blood pressure, atheroma, and to maintain cardiovascular health
+ With barberry and echinacea to treat bacterial and fungal infections

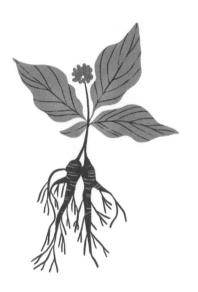

Korean ginseng

Panax ginseng

In traditional Chinese medicine, ginseng supports vitality, calms the spirit, and aids yin-deficient states, where the body's reserves and capacity to self-repair has been compromised. In young people ginseng is tonic and stimulant – take short term to promote mental and physical performance and improve stamina. In older adults, it acts as a restorative medicine, supporting energy levels, countering age-related ill health, and improving resilience and immune function. Hormonally active, ginseng helps to improve libido in both men and women.

PARTS USED
Root

MAIN USES
Chronic stress and fatigue, menopausal tonic, low libido, erectile dysfunction, to improve physical and mental performance, to maintain health in later years

MAIN ACTIONS
Adaptogen, tonic, antiageing, anti-inflammatory, immune tonic

BEST TAKEN AS
Internal use
+ Tincture, powder, concentrated extracts

DOSAGE
Internal use
+ Tincture 2.5 ml (½ tsp) one to three time a day
+ Powder 0.5–2.5 g (⅛–½ tsp) a day; start low and increase dosage gradually

LENGTH OF TREATMENT
Healthy young adults can take this for up to three months at a time. In chronic fatigue and for adults aged 60+, low-dose long-term treatment is recommended.

CAUTIONS
Do not take ginseng during pregnancy. Excessive doses can cause sleep disturbance and high blood pressure. Avoid caffeine when taking ginseng. Ginseng can be too stimulant for sensitive people (try maca instead).

COMBINATIONS
+ With ashwagandha for nervous exhaustion and chronic fatigue
+ With St John's wort and black cohosh for menopausal tiredness and hot flushing

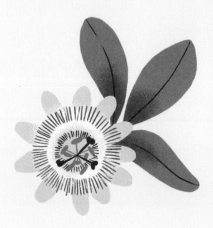

Passion flower

Passiflora incarnata

Passion flower has a tranquilizing effect on the nervous system, reducing overactivity and associated tension. It is ideal for anxiety, inability to relax, and states of extreme apprehension – take in small repeated doses. Commonly used to aid sleep, it works best when first getting off to sleep; for frequent waking take it with valerian. The herb's sedative and relaxant activity works well in reducing high blood pressure and palpitations caused by distress. Passion flower's analgesic activity can prove useful in headache, toothache, muscle pains, and so on.

PARTS USED
Leaf

MAIN USES
Insomnia, anxiety and nervous irritability, headache, pain, high blood pressure

MAIN ACTIONS
Sedative, tranquilizing, antispasmodic, mild analgesic

BEST TAKEN AS
Internal use
+ Infusion, tincture, concentrated extracts

DOSAGE
Internal use
+ Infusion 5 g (2½ tsp) dried leaf to 200 ml (7 fl oz) water a day
+ Tincture 2.5 ml (½ tsp) one to four times a day

LENGTH OF TREATMENT
Long-term treatment at a low dose is fine.

CAUTIONS
Large doses of passion flower can cause drowsiness. Do not take high doses in pregnancy.

COMBINATIONS
+ With Californian poppy or valerian to aid sleep and relieve anxiety
+ With chamomile and cramp bark for neck ache, muscle cramps, and spasmodic pain

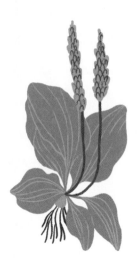

Plantain

Plantago major, P. lanceolata

A potent wound healer with a mix of astringent and demulcent constituents, plantain has a particular application in healing inflamed and damaged mucous membranes. An infusion will help soothe dry or inflamed mucous membranes in the nose and throat, moistening the passageways or reducing excess mucus production. It is equally useful within the digestive tract taken in combination with other herbs in acid indigestion and reflux and will support large bowel health, potentially helping to treat leaky gut syndrome.

PARTS USED
Aerial parts

MAIN USES
Excess mucus production, dry mucous membranes, hay fever, hoarseness, upper respiratory tract infection, gastritis, diarrhoea, irritable bowel syndrome; topically, heals wounds, haemorrhoids, and ulcers

MAIN ACTIONS
Wound healer, anticatarrhal, diuretic, expectorant, antiviral

BEST TAKEN AS
Internal use
+ Infusion, tincture
External use
+ Cream, ointment

DOSAGE
Internal use
+ Infusion up to 10 g (⅓ oz) dried herb to 200 ml (7 fl oz) water a day
+ Tincture 5 ml (1 tsp) one to three times a day
External use
+ Cream, ointment, as wanted

LENGTH OF TREATMENT
Long-term treatment at a low dose is fine.

CAUTIONS
Plantain is a safe herb.

COMBINATIONS
+ With chia or flaxseed for dry cough, sore throat, and hoarseness
+ With yarrow to support tissue repair (bruises, fractures, and to aid wound healing)

Propolis

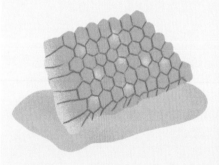

Propolis is a bee product derived from flowers, buds, and gums of plants and trees. Though not a herb, it is included in this book because it is an exceptionally useful natural medicine. Propolis is a powerful antiseptic with major antibacterial activity. Diluted tincture makes an effective wash to cleanse wounds and prevent infection (it will sting!). Taken internally, propolis has an affinity with the upper respiratory tract and can be taken diluted and sweetened with honey for colds, flu, coughs, sore throat, and chesty conditions.

PARTS USED
All

MAIN USES
Respiratory and digestive infections, chronic infections, to clean wounds and aid healing

MAIN ACTIONS
Antimicrobial, immune tonic, anti-inflammatory, wound healing

BEST TAKEN AS
Internal use
+ Tincture, concentrated extracts

DOSAGE
Internal use
+ Tincture 10 drops of 1:20 extract up to four times a day (concentrations vary greatly, so adjust dosage accordingly)

LENGTH OF TREATMENT
Short-term treatment is recommended.

CAUTIONS
Propolis is known to cause allergic reactions, so do a skin test first. Do not take if you have kidney disease.

COMBINATIONS
+ With elderberry and/or echinacea in upper respiratory tract infection
+ With liquorice to treat mouth ulcers, sore tongue, and toothache

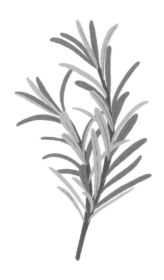

Rosemary

Rosmarinus officinalis

A much-loved garden herb, rosemary protects and restores in equal measure. It enhances memory and concentration and protects the nervous system from inflammatory damage. It has been used by students preparing for exams for at least two thousand years. Current research suggests that small doses are more effective than large ones ("less" can be "more" in herbal medicine) – eating a small sprig of fresh rosemary leaves a day is thought to aid the body in resisting a range of processes associated with ageing.

PARTS USED
Aerial parts

MAIN USES
Nervous exhaustion, chronic stress, lowered mood, mild to moderate depression, low blood pressure, failure to thrive (weak digestion and dizziness), as aid to memory and cognition, to reduce risk of sunburn, as a restorative and to slow ageing processes.

MAIN ACTIONS
Neuroprotective, antidepressant, anti-inflammatory, bitter tonic, circulatory stimulant, antiageing, protects against sunburn

BEST TAKEN AS
Internal use
+ Fresh leaf infusion, tincture, powder
External use
+ Infusion as hair tonic (massage well into scalp), essential oil

DOSAGE
Internal use
+ Fresh leaf 1 small sprig once or twice a day
+ Dried leaf or powder up to 5 g (2½ tsp) a day
+ Infusion 5 g (2½ tsp) dried herb to 200 ml (7 fl oz) water a day
+ Tincture 2.5 ml (½ tsp) up to three times a day
External use
+ Essential oil 5 per cent dilution in carrier oil

LENGTH OF TREATMENT
As a one-off before exams and presentations. Long-term use is safe at 1–2.5 g (¼ –½ tsp) a day.

CAUTIONS
Do not take essential oil internally.

COMBINATIONS
+ With lemon balm to aid memory and cognition
+ With St John's wort for mild to moderate depression

Chia

Salvia hispanica

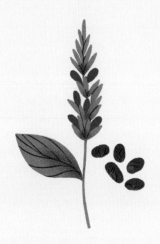

With a high essential fatty acid and fibre content, chia seed is both a nutritious food and a valued medicine. Looking a bit like frogspawn when soaked in water, chia's gooey, mucilaginous consistency makes it a soothing remedy for dry mouth, sore throat, and dry irritable coughs. The seeds work as a prebiotic within the gut, promoting a healthy gut flora, slowing the absorption of fats and sugars, and maintaining regular bowel movements. Chia is oestrogenic and makes a useful supplement during perimenopause and the menopause.

PARTS USED
Seed

MAIN USES
Dry mouth, sore throat, dry coughs, as a bulk laxative, as a prebiotic, as a perimenopausal and menopausal supplement

MAIN ACTIONS
Demulcent, emollient, oestrogenic

BEST TAKEN AS
Internal use
+ Seeds soaked in water

DOSAGE
Internal use
+ Seeds up to 25 g (1 oz) a day, soaked in 125 ml (4 fl oz) water and blended in a smoothie; enables absorption of omega-3 oils (Seeds need to be ground to release omega-3 oils)

LENGTH OF TREATMENT
Long-term treatment at a low dose is fine.

CAUTIONS
Excess intake of chia can cause digestive symptoms. Once ground, store in a closed container in the fridge and consume within two days, as omega-3 oils go rancid very quickly.

COMBINATIONS
+ With black cohosh and St John's wort for menopausal symptoms
+ With artichoke and/or dandelion to control raised cholesterol levels

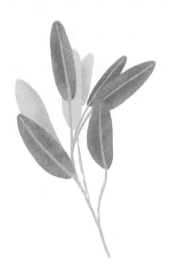

Sage

Salvia officinalis

Sage can help in treating many complaints. Use an infusion as a gargle or mouthwash for sore throat, sore tongue, and mouth ulcers, to reduce excess catarrh, counter infection, and to relieve diarrhoea. Fresh leaves or essential oil make a good insect repellent. Sage is known to support memory and healthy cognitive function and may protect against neurodegenerative diseases, such as dementia. A key remedy for menopausal symptoms, sage infusion or tincture can be helpful in easing "brain fog" and aiding memory and concentration.

PARTS USED
Leaf

MAIN USES
Mouth ulcers, sore throat, excess catarrh, perimenopausal and menopausal symptoms (especially hot flushing and sweats), poor memory/cognition, breast engorgement; to aid weaning

MAIN ACTIONS
Astringent, antiseptic, tonic, reduces sweating, oestrogenic, neuroprotective, digestive tonic

BEST TAKEN AS
Internal use
+ Infusion, tincture

DOSAGE
Internal use
+ Infusion 5 g (2½ tsp) dried herb to 200 ml (7 fl oz) water a day
+ Tincture 2.5 ml (½ tsp) one to three times a day

LENGTH OF TREATMENT
Long-term treatment at a low dose is fine.

CAUTIONS
Do not take sage essential oil internally. Do not take during pregnancy or while breastfeeding (except when weaning). Excessive doses can be toxic.

COMBINATIONS
+ With plantain for sore throat and hoarseness
+ With liquorice and/or black cohosh for hot flushing and night sweats

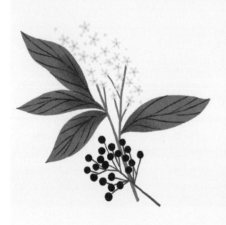

Elder

Sambucus nigra

Elderberry has significant antiviral activity and is popular for colds and flu, possibly being helpful in Covid-19, where it appears to support immune function and improve recovery time. Berry and flower can be used to treat upper respiratory complaints, the flowers having a stronger, drying effect on mucous membranes and proving helpful in excess mucus production. The flowers are diaphoretic and an infusion helps relieve feverish states. Carefully strained, an infusion makes a good eyewash for sore and tired eyes.

PARTS USED
Flower, berry

MAIN USES
Colds, flu, upper respiratory complaints (including nasal congestion, sinusitis, allergic rhinitis, and catarrhal headache), sore, inflamed eyes, conjunctivitis

MAIN ACTIONS
Anticatarrhal, increases sweating, antiviral, anti-inflammatory, mild diuretic

BEST TAKEN AS
Internal use
+ Infusion, tincture, powder, concentrated extracts

DOSAGE
Internal use
+ Infusion 10 g (⅓ oz) flower or berry to 200 ml (7 fl oz) water a day
+ Tincture 5 ml (1 tsp) one to three times a day
+ Powder 2.5–7.5 g (½–1½ tsp) a day

LENGTH OF TREATMENT
Long-term treatment at a low dose is fine.

CAUTIONS
Do not consume unripe (green) elderberries, as they are potentially toxic.

COMBINATIONS
+ Elderflower with chamomile and plantain for watery catarrhal problems/rhinitis, including hay fever
+ Elderberry with echinacea and propolis for upper respiratory infections

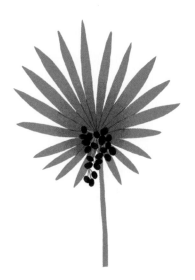

Saw palmetto

Serenoa repens

Saw palmetto's hormonal activity makes it a key soothing and relaxing remedy for problems affecting the urinary tract. With anabolic, muscle-building activity it can be taken to improve muscle bulk and strength in the older person and after prolonged illness. In men, it counters the hormonal imbalance that causes benign prostatic hypertrophy (BPH). It can prove highly effective in relieving BPH symptoms and easing related problems such as pain on urination, poor flow, urgency, and frequency.

PARTS USED
Berry

MAIN USES
Low libido, enlarged prostate, prostatitis, irritable bladder, erectile dysfunction, lower urinary tract problems such as poor flow and frequency

MAIN ACTIONS
Endocrine agent, anabolic, anti-inflammatory, antispasmodic, diuretic, mild sedative

BEST TAKEN AS
Internal use
+ Tincture, concentrated extracts

DOSAGE
Internal use
+ Tincture 2.5 ml (½ tsp) one to three times a day
+ Concentrated extract

LENGTH OF TREATMENT
Best taken as concentrated extracts, long-term treatment at a low dose is fine.

CAUTIONS
Saw palmetto can cause digestive symptoms. Do not use during pregnancy, while breast-feeding, if taking prescribed hormonal drugs, or if you have a hormone-dependent cancer.

COMBINATIONS
+ With ashwagandha and ginkgo for low libido in both women and men, and for erectile dysfunction
+ With horsetail and nettle root for enlarged prostate and lower urinary tract problems, including frequency and discomfort

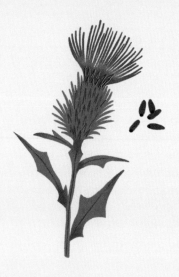

Milk thistle

Silybum marianum

Milk thistle is a key medicine for the liver, promoting its ability to detoxify and to protect itself from toxicity. It will often normalize raised liver enzymes, where no underlying pathology has been found. It is the go-to medicine for liver disorders associated with obesity, notably fatty liver disease, and it will aid in the process of shedding weight. Its powerful, antioxidant activity makes it an easily consumed antiageing remedy, countering the inflammatory processes that lie behind many chronic health conditions.

PARTS USED
Seed

MAIN USES
Liver disorders (fatty liver, poor liver function), weight loss, clearing toxins and waste products, inflammatory skin conditions

MAIN ACTIONS
Liver protective, stimulates breast milk, antioxidant, antitoxin, anticancer

BEST TAKEN AS
Internal use
+ Ground seeds, concentrated extracts

DOSAGE
Internal use
+ Ground seed 2.5–5 g (1–2 tsp) a day
+ Concentrated extracts (140 mg silymarin) 1–2 times a day

LENGTH OF TREATMENT
Seeds can be taken as a food supplement.

CAUTIONS
A safe herb, milk thistle may cause allergic reactions, though rarely. Store freshly ground seeds in a closed container in a fridge for up to two days.

COMBINATIONS
+ With artichoke for fatty liver disease, to aid weight loss, and to lower cholesterol levels
+ With ginger and turmeric for chronic inflammatory diseases such as rheumatoid arthritis and psoriasis

Comfrey

Symphytum officinale

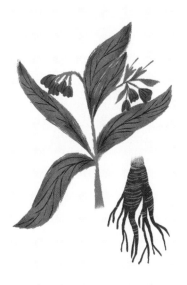

Comfrey can be highly effective in promoting tissue repair and makes a perfect first-aid remedy for sprains and bruises. When applied as soon as possible after an accident or operation – for example, on a sprained ankle or on the cheek after a tooth extraction – it prevents inflammatory damage spreading further than necessary and speeds up the rate of tissue healing. The infused oil can be used as a base to carry essential oils to soothe and relieve local joint pain and inflammation. The ointment or cream can be used on any skin blemish that requires healing.

PARTS USED
Root, leaf

MAIN USES
Bruises and sprains, fractures and broken bones, arthritic joints, scars, inflammatory skin conditions, acne

MAIN ACTIONS
Tissue healer, astringent, anti-inflammatory, demulcent, emollient

BEST TAKEN AS
External use
+ Infused oil, cream, ointment, lotion

DOSAGE
External use
+ Infused oil, cream, ointment, lotion apply one to three times a day to affected tissue

LENGTH OF TREATMENT
Topical use for up to three months – for example, to aid scar healing.

CAUTIONS
Do not take comfrey internally. Apply only to unbroken skin. Do not use it on broken bones until the bone has been set.

COMBINATIONS
+ With chamomile cream and witch hazel water for inflammatory skin problems such as eczema
+ With *gotu kola* tincture or concentrated extracts to promote tissue healing (comfrey topically, *gotu kola* internally)

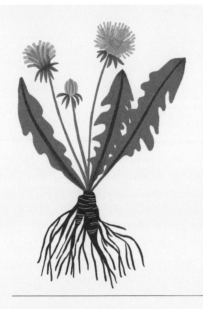

Dandelion

Taraxacum officinale

An instantly recognizable garden "weed" with its yellow sun-bright flowers, dandelion is a gentle and effective herbal medicine. Safe for children, dandelion root makes an excellent detox remedy for skin conditions such as acne and eczema and, with echinacea, in chronic skin infections. The leaf is diuretic and powerfully increases urine output, therefore is helpful in treating fluid retention and "boggy" conditions associated with arthritis or poor circulation. It is commonly used alongside other remedies to treat high blood pressure.

PARTS USED
Leaf, root

MAIN USES
Fluid retention, high blood pressure (leaf), abdominal bloating, skin disorders, chronic constipation, metabolic problems (including pre-diabetes), anticancer (root)

MAIN ACTIONS
Bitter, diuretic, detoxifying agent

BEST TAKEN AS
Internal use
+ Leaf: infusion, tincture, powder
+ Root: decoction, tincture, powder

DOSAGE
Internal use
+ Leaf infusion 2.5–10 g (1–5 tsp) dried leaf to 200 ml (7 fl oz) water a day
+ Leaf tincture 5 ml (1 tsp) three times a day
+ Leaf powder 2.5–10 g (½–2 tsp) a day
+ Root decoction 2.5–7.5 g (1–3 tsp) root to 300 ml (10½ fl oz) water a day
+ Root tincture 5 ml (1 tsp) three times a day
+ Root powder 2.5–7.5 g (½–1½ tsp) a day

LENGTH OF TREATMENT
Low doses can be taken indefinitely; doses above 5 g (1 tsp) powder or 10 ml (2 tsp) tincture a day should be taken for one to two months only.

CAUTIONS
To treat toxic states such as inflammatory skin problems, start with a low dose and increase slowly. Dandelion can cause allergic reactions, though this is rare.

COMBINATIONS
+ Leaf with hawthorn and garlic for high blood pressure
+ Root with marigold and echinacea to support detox and in skin disorders

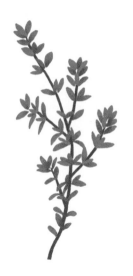

Thyme

Thymus vulgaris

Gentle acting but potent, thyme is a safe remedy for children. It has an enlivening effect on the body, improving its ability to resist infection – especially viral and fungal infection and to cope with ongoing stress. Sweetened with honey, an infusion or tincture makes an effective remedy for coughs and chesty conditions – its essential oil (removed from the body via the lungs) has a directly antiseptic activity within the respiratory airways. An infusion can be used as a wash on infected skin, especially for fungal problems, and as a hair tonic.

PARTS USED
Aerial parts

MAIN USES
Cough and chest infections, wheeziness, fungal infections, threadworm; topically, to treat bites and stings, rheumatic aches and pains, fungal infections, and as a hair tonic

MAIN ACTIONS
Antimicrobial, tonic, antispasmodic, expectorant, expels worms

BEST TAKEN AS
Internal use
+ Infusion, tincture, concentrated extracts
External use
+ Essential oil

DOSAGE
Internal use
+ Infusion 5 g (2½ tsp) dried herb to 200 ml (7 fl oz) water a day; tincture 2.5 ml (½ tsp) one to three times a day
External use
+ Essential oil, diluted: max. 5 per cent dilution in carrier oil

LENGTH OF TREATMENT
Long-term treatment at a low dose is fine.

CAUTIONS
Thyme can cause allergic reactions, although this is rare. Do not take thyme essential oil internally.

COMBINATIONS
+ With elecampane and garlic for coughs, wheeziness, and bronchitis
+ With rosemary applied to the scalp to treat hair loss; use as a final rinse and then massage into the scalp

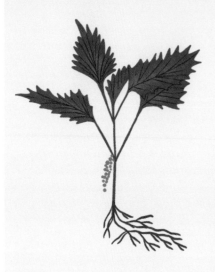

Nettle

Urtica dioica

Nettle leaf is highly nutritious and aids detoxification, increasing urine output and the elimination of waste products. Taken long-term it is therefore valuable in arthritic conditions, such as arthritis and gout, as well as osteoporosis, countering inflammation and encouraging tissue repair. The leaf often proves useful in treating allergic conditions like "nettle" rash (urticaria), eczema, and hay fever, and in skin problems such as acne, eczema, and psoriasis. The root is a useful alternative to saw palmetto in treating an enlarged prostate.

PARTS USED
Leaf, root

MAIN USES
Arthritis, gout, osteoporosis, nosebleeds, heavy menstrual bleeding, allergies (including nettle rash and hay fever), skin problems, enlarged prostate, prostatitis (root), to prevent kidney stones

MAIN ACTIONS
Tonic, anti-inflammatory, antiallergenic, diuretic, antidiabetic, staunches bleeding, increases breast milk levels, endocrine agent (root)

BEST TAKEN AS
Internal use
+ Infusion, decoction, tincture, powder, concentrated extracts
+ The fresh plant tops can be eaten as a nutritious vegetable

DOSAGE
Internal use
+ Infusion 10 g (⅓ oz) dried leaf to 200 ml (7 fl oz) water a day
+ Decoction 10 g (⅓ oz) root to 300 ml (10½ fl oz) water a day
+ Tincture 5 ml (1 tsp) one to three times a day
+ Powder up to 7.5 g (1½ tsp) a day

LENGTH OF TREATMENT
Long-term treatment is fine.

CAUTIONS
None known. Nettles sting, so wear gloves when picking them fresh!

COMBINATIONS
+ With black cohosh and horsetail for osteoporosis
+ With ginger and turmeric for arthritis, rheumatic disease, and gout

Valerian

Valeriana officinalis

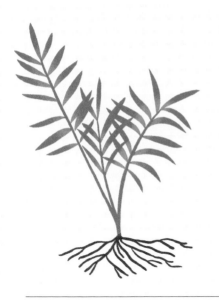

Safe and non-addictive, valerian is a calming and tranquilizing remedy, helpful in almost all cases of panic and anxiety, slowing nervous activity and breathing, and relaxing tensed muscles. It can be of great value for chronic "worriers". Most complaints involving tension will benefit from valerian's muscle-relaxant effect, making the herb useful in situations as varied as digestive cramps, tight-chestedness, frozen shoulder, back pain, and neck tension. Valerian helps with insomnia and in sleep difficulty related to anxiety and stress.

PARTS USED
Root

MAIN USES
Stress, anxiety, inability to relax, nervous tension, panic attacks, poor sleep, muscle tension, menstrual cramps, irritable bowel syndrome, high blood pressure

MAIN ACTIONS
Relaxant, sedative, antianxiety, antispasmodic, sleep aid, lowers blood pressure

BEST TAKEN AS
Internal use
+ Tincture, concentrated extracts

DOSAGE
Internal use
+ Tincture 2.5 ml (½ tsp) up to four times a day or 20 drops/1 ml (¼ tsp) up to ten times a day
+ Powder up to 3 g (½ tsp) a day
+ Concentrated extract

LENGTH OF TREATMENT
Long-term treatment is fine.

CAUTIONS
Sensitivity to valerian varies greatly. In some people it causes excess stimulation. Start with a low dose and increase as needed. Excess doses cause drowsiness.

COMBINATIONS
+ With passion flower and rosemary for chronic stress, anxiety, and nervous exhaustion
+ With cramp bark for muscle aches and pains throughout the body

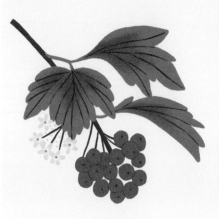

Cramp bark

Viburnum opulus

Cramp bark is a safe and effective antispasmodic, useful in almost any condition where overtight muscles are present. This makes it a key remedy for rheumatic and muscular aches and pains, including strained and tired muscles after sports activities. It can be very helpful in backache involving muscle spasms and is worth trying to relieve almost any type of cramping. Though this is mainly a treatment for physical tension, it fits well alongside relaxant herbs such as St John's wort and valerian in relieving muscle tension from anxiety.

PARTS USED
Root

MAIN USES
Muscle tension and spasm, arthritic pain and stiffness, backache, asthma, menstrual cramps, high blood pressure

MAIN ACTIONS
Antispasmodic, lowers blood pressure, relaxant, mildly sedative

BEST TAKEN AS
Internal use
+ Decoction, tincture, powder, concentrated extracts
External use
+ Decoction, tincture

DOSAGE
Internal use
+ Decoction 5–10 g (2½–5 tsp) dried root to 300 ml (10½ fl oz) water a day
+ Tincture 2.5 ml (½ tsp) one to four times a day
+ Powdered root up to 2.5 g (½ tsp) a day
External use
+ The decoction or diluted tincture can be applied as a compress to soothe sore, tense muscles

LENGTH OF TREATMENT
Long-term treatment at a low dose is fine.

CAUTIONS
Cramp bark is a safe herb.

COMBINATIONS
+ With valerian for muscle pain and cramps, especially if associated with anxiety and tension
+ With hawthorn and garlic for high blood pressure

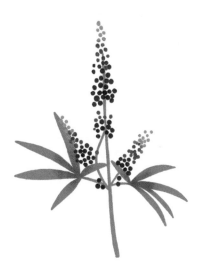

Chaste tree

Vitex agnus-castus

Chaste tree acts on the hypothalamus at the base of the brain and promotes dopamine and melatonin release. This can lead to increased progesterone secretion by the ovaries, though the herb appears to aid balanced hormone levels through the menstrual cycle, rather than to selectively increase progesterone levels. It finds use in any situation involving menstrual irregularity, including pre-menstrual syndrome. It is a key remedy in perimenopausal conditions and, as it lowers testosterone levels, is useful when trying to clear acne.

PARTS USED
Berry

MAIN USES
Pre-menstrual syndrome, breast tenderness, infertility, menopausal symptoms, irregular and disturbed sleep, acne; to regulate the menstrual cycle

MAIN ACTIONS
Hormone balancer, progesterogenic, stimulates breast milk, aids sleep

BEST TAKEN AS
Internal use
+ Tincture, capsules, concentrated extracts

DOSAGE
Internal use
+ Tincture 20–30 drops tincture on waking each morning

LENGTH OF TREATMENT
Usually needs to be taken regularly for a minimum of three months.

CAUTIONS
Avoid chaste tree during pregnancy. Concurrent use with the contraceptive pill is not advisable.

COMBINATIONS
+ With black cohosh to promote hormonal balance and for pre-menstrual syndrome including menstrual headaches and breast tenderness
+ With marigold, echinacea, and yellow dock for acne

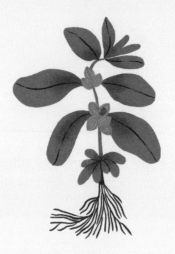

Ashwagandha

Withania somnifera

A key remedy for long-term stress and chronic infection, ashwagandha is a well-tolerated, gentle-acting adaptogen that supports and strengthens cognitive performance, invigorates the body and its capacity to cope with stress, and strengthens immune function. A safe herb, it is thought to be suitable for older children. Ashwagandha is anti-inflammatory and can be taken to relieve arthritic aches and pains and to promote tissue healing. Other uses include to support male and female fertility and as adjunctive treatment in cancer.

PARTS USED
Root

MAIN USES
Chronic stress, chronic fatigue, anxiety, lowered immune function and chronic infection, insomnia (especially where anxiety and stress are factors), male and female infertility

MAIN ACTIONS
Adaptogen, anti-inflammatory, tonic, immune support, promotes sleep quality, increases libido and fertility

BEST TAKEN AS
Internal use
+ Tincture, powder, concentrated extracts

DOSAGE
Internal use
+ Tincture 2–10 ml (up to 2 tsp) a day
+ Powder 2–6 g (½–1 tsp) a day as divided doses

LENGTH OF TREATMENT
Medium- to long-term use is recommended for chronic conditions.

CAUTIONS
Avoid during pregnancy as its safety is unconfirmed.

COMBINATIONS
+ With echinacea and turmeric to aid recovery from infection, including flu and Covid-19
+ With passion flower and valerian for anxiety, nervous exhaustion, and insomnia

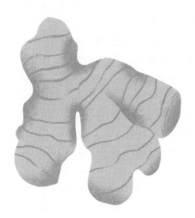

Ginger

Zingiber officinale

Ginger has long been prized for its warming, invigorating action, relieving chills and supporting healthy circulation. Whether taken on its own or combined with garlic and cinnamon, its makes an excellent first-aid treatment for viral infections of all kinds. A go-to remedy for many digestive problems, an infusion of fresh ginger root will ease and bring relief to symptoms such as nausea, travel sickness, stomach ache, and indigestion.

PARTS USED
Root

MAIN USES
Colds, flu, fever, nausea, travel sickness, vomiting and indigestion, poor peripheral circulation (including chilblains), headache and migraine, arthritis

MAIN ACTIONS
Warming digestive tonic, circulatory stimulant, antiemetic, relieves wind and bloating, anti-inflammatory, antiviral, antimicrobial

BEST TAKEN AS
Internal use
+ Infusion, tincture, concentrated extracts
External use
+ Juice, essential oil

DOSAGE
Internal use
+ Infusion 5 g (1 tsp) fresh root or 2 g (½ tsp) dry root in 200 ml (7 fl oz) water a day
+ Tincture up to 3 ml (½ tsp) a day
External use
+ Juice, squeeze fresh root in garlic crusher and apply to cold sores and chilblains
+ Essential oil dilute 5 drops in 20 drops carrier oil and massage in to ease joint and muscle aches and pains

LENGTH OF TREATMENT
Long-term treatment is fine.

CAUTIONS
Do not take essential oil internally. Do not take if you are suffering from peptic ulcers.

COMBINATIONS
+ With chamomile and fennel in nausea and travel sickness
+ With nettle leaf and turmeric for arthritic pain and inflammation

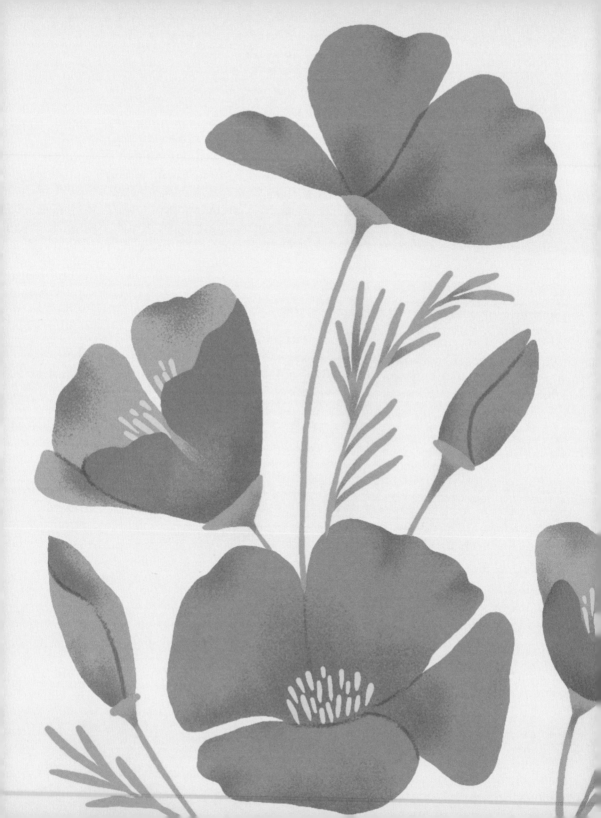

Using Herbal Medicines Wisely

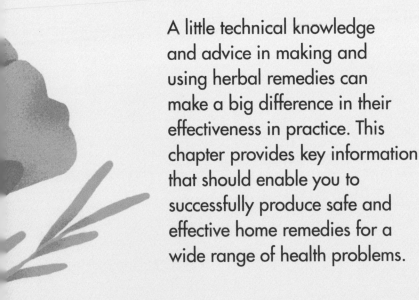

A little technical knowledge and advice in making and using herbal remedies can make a big difference in their effectiveness in practice. This chapter provides key information that should enable you to successfully produce safe and effective home remedies for a wide range of health problems.

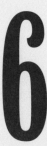

Herbs for Everyday Living

Working with herbal medicines is not too different from cooking, and many of the skills needed to use herbs successfully are similar to those used every day in the kitchen. Herbs and spices can be confusing because they are both foods, belonging to the kitchen, and medicines, belonging to the dispensary. There are no concerns about chopping up fresh garlic and ginger to add to a stew, but a different set of rules applies when these foods are to be used as medicines.

Some restaurants in China offer a "medicinal food" menu on which portions of Chinese angelica, ginger, or ginseng root, among many other herbal ingredients, are served with selected meals. This is one way of ensuring that a meal is nutritious and directly therapeutic. Including herbs in your everyday life in this way – in cooking, as smoothies, infusions, and supplements – is much the best way to use them. In doing this, you are using herbs to keep healthy rather than simply resorting to them when you get ill.

There will also be times when you want to take herbal remedies as medicines or to relieve unwanted symptoms and treat ill health. In such cases, you need to use herbs thoughtfully and with respect. This section of the book aims to help you feel confident about developing the skills needed to use herbal medicines in this way.

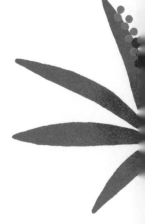

DECIDING WHICH HERBS TO USE

When using herbs medicinally, it is important to choose the right herbs at the right dosage and in the most suitable form. Accurately targeted herbs can make the difference between successful recovery and no change at all. The following pages offer advice on understanding a herb's actions and indications, on dosage, and on buying herbs. At the end of the section, you will find information on cautions.

Every time you consider turning to a herbal remedy, working through the following process will help you choose the most appropriate herbs.

1. Decide what the main symptoms are. If there are several, rank them in order of importance.

2. Make a list of herbs that are known to help relieve or treat these symptoms. As far as possible, choose herbs with actions that will treat several symptoms at the same time.

3. Select two to three herbs from this list, ideally the ones that are most likely to be helpful when taken together.

4. Work out how you are going to take them: as infusions, tinctures, or concentrated extracts, and so on.

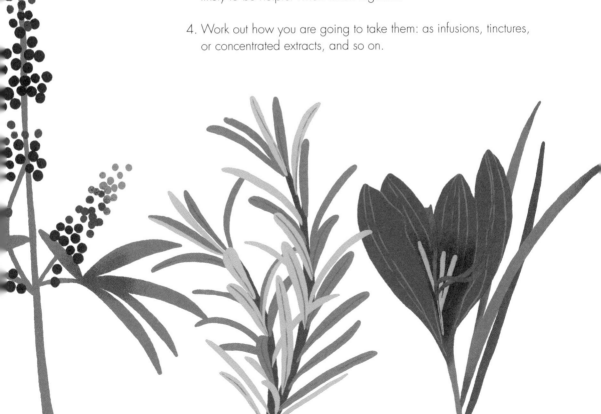

DOSAGE

If you have ever eaten too hot a curry, you will have experienced the effect of overdosing on hot spices such as chilli and black pepper. Creating a curry that warms and has a bit of fire, but does not burn, is a good way of describing what a correct dose is in herbal medicine. When it comes to dosage, it is best to be cautious rather than over-enthusiastic, at least to begin with. As with spices in a curry, once you have some experience in using a herb, you can be more creative in combining it with other herbs and selecting appropriate dosages.

General guidelines for dosage are given in the box on the opposite page. For the herb profiles in Chapter 5, the dosages given are recommended maximums. "More" does not mean "better" in herbal medicine, and in some cases, increasing the dosage actually reduces the therapeutic effect of a herb. Always check the dosage given for a herb before using it.

HOW LONG SHOULD I TAKE THE REMEDY?

There are no simple rules that answer this question. The most useful generalization is that acute complaints need short-term treatment and chronic complaints need long-term treatment. If you suddenly develop inflamed, itchy skin on your wrists and this has not happened before, applying a suitable cream is likely to heal the skin within a matter of days; however, if you are prone to this problem, and for example have a history of eczema, longer-term treatment will be needed. Whether symptoms clear quickly or not, it always makes sense to continue with the remedies for a few extra days or weeks. Stopping too quickly increases the risk that symptoms will recur. When taking herbs to maintain health, to slow ageing, or to prevent illness, it is best to take a low to moderate dose long term.

STANDARD DOSES

+ **Infusions** Whether you are using a single herb or a mixture of herbs, the standard recommended dose for an infusion is 10 g dried herb or 15 g fresh herb to 200 ml water (⅓ oz dried herb or ½ oz fresh herb to 7 fl oz water), taken in divided doses through the day. Herbs such as sage and yarrow are strong acting and quantities should be halved for the same volume of water.

+ **Decoctions** For decoctions, use the same quantity of herb as for an infusion (see above), but with 300 ml (10½ fl oz) water. On being simmered for 20 minutes, about 200 ml (7 fl oz) liquid will remain.

+ **Tinctures** The standard dose for a single herb is 5 ml (1 tsp) twice a day or 2.5 ml (½ tsp) four times a day. Two or more herbs combined can usually be taken at 5 ml (1 tsp) three times a day.

+ **Powders** There is no standard dose for powders. Follow the recommended doses in the herb profiles.

+ **Concentrated extracts** Take these according to the manufacturer's recommendations or as prescribed by a healthcare practitioner.

+ See also, recommended dosages for Pregnancy and Breastfeeding (pp. 145–147) and for Children (p. 157)

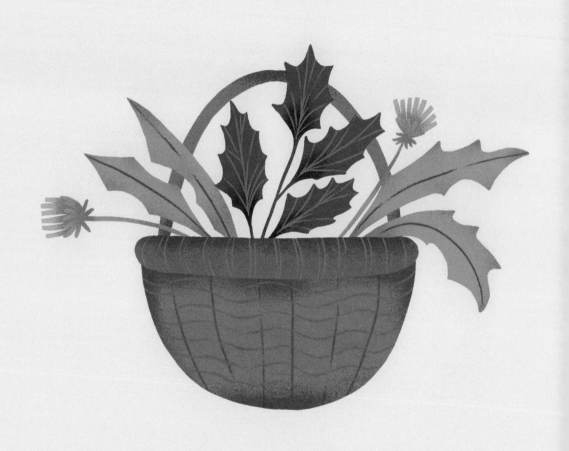

SOURCING HERBS

All reputable suppliers and manufacturers of herbal medicines apply quality control to ensure that they start with the correct herbal material of the right quality. Quality is essential in herbal medicine – old or poor-quality herbal material will have inferior or non-existent medicinal activity. Adulteration, where inferior quality material or foreign substances are added to the correct herbal material, is not a rare event and is particularly common in powdered herbs such as turmeric. Chalk, dyes, and rice powder are some of the adulterants used. When buying dried herbs and powders, buy from a well-known, established herbal supplier and check use-by dates.

HOW CAN I KEEP COSTS DOWN?

Herbal remedies are usually reasonably priced, but when long-term treatment is needed, cost can become an important factor. The most economic way of using herbs is to grow your own: echinacea, garlic, lemon balm, rosemary, and sage, to name but a few, can be grown in most temperate regions. You can gather plants such as dandelion and nettle from the wild. Unprocessed dried herbs and powders are often the next most cost-effective remedies, but this is not always the case. For example, taking 5 g (2½ tsp) of dried herb a day as an infusion can be more expensive than 15 ml (1 tbsp) of tincture. Check prices and compare them. Tinctures and concentrated extracts in tablet or capsule form can sometimes be better value, as they have a long shelf life.

Bear in mind that alongside cost-effectiveness lies convenience and compliance – for example, it is a false economy to buy dried herbs because they are cheaper, if for one reason or another you fail to take them regularly. If you do not have the time to make your own preparations, take powders, tinctures, tablets, or capsules.

ACCURATE IDENTIFICATION

Usually, when you buy herbs or manufactured herbal products in a health store or online, there is no need to worry, as the necessary checks will have been made to ensure they have been identified correctly. If you are harvesting herbs from your garden or from the wild, you must be certain what herb you are collecting. Correct identification is essential. For example, ragwort (*Senecio jacobaea*), which is toxic to the liver, can easily be mistaken for St John's wort: both grow on waste ground, are roughly the same height, and produce clusters of bright yellow flowers in the summer.

CAUTIONS

For best results, and to avoid unwanted effects, herbal medicines need to be used with care. As with all medicines, herbal remedies can sometimes cause side-effects, provoke allergic reactions, or interact harmfully with prescribed medication. Make sure to read the listed cautions before taking a herb.

SIDE-EFFECTS

Taking excessive doses of any medicine, herbal or conventional, can produce side-effects. By and large, herbal medicines are extremely safe and side-effects are rare. However, unwanted symptoms do occur. It is important to be alert to this possibility, especially if you are taking a herbal remedy for the first time. Side-effects produced by herbs typically involve minor symptoms such as digestive upsets and headaches. Sometimes existing symptoms can flare up when you start taking a new remedy. In either case, if you suspect that you are reacting badly to a herbal remedy, stop taking it. If symptoms are minor, try an alternative remedy. If they are severe, or continue to worsen, seek immediate advice from your healthcare practitioner.

PRE-EXISTING HEALTH CONDITIONS

Some herbal medicines need to be avoided by those who have certain pre-existing health conditions, as they may worsen symptoms. For example, people with high blood pressure should not take liquorice, as its action on the adrenal glands can further raise blood pressure. Before taking a herbal remedy, check the cautions listed in each herb profile, to ensure that it will be safer for you to take.

SERIOUS ILLNESS

If you have any of the "red flag" conditions listed on pp. 22–23, get immediate medical attention. See also, Consulting a Herbal Practitioner, p. 246.

INTERACTIONS WITH PRESCRIBED MEDICINES	If you are taking prescribed medication, it makes sense to let your doctor know if you plan to take herbal medicines. It works the other way, too – if you see a herbal practitioner, keep them informed if you are taking prescribed medication. The 50 herbs covered in this book are mostly safe to take alongside prescribed medicines at the recommended dosage. However, some herbs influence the effects of prescribed medicines, interacting with them and increasing or decreasing their strength of action. Foods are as much an issue with respect to interactions as herbs. For example, grapefruit potentiates the action of statins, while many foodstuffs, such as grapes, red wine, and mushrooms, affect liver enzyme levels and rates of drug metabolism. Often these interactions are slight and, in some cases, they are beneficial: milk thistle is thought to enhance the effectiveness of chemotherapy in certain cancers, for example. However, herb–drug interactions can cause serious, life-threatening problems. The main herb of concern here is St John's wort. Though very safe as a medicine, it interacts with a range of prescribed medicines and speeds up their breakdown within the body. If you are taking prescribed medication and plan to take herbal remedies (especially St John's wort), always check first with a herbal practitioner or your doctor.
SENSITIVITY TO MEDICINES	If you know that you, or someone you are giving herbs to, is sensitive to medicines, it is a good policy to start new herbal remedies by taking a small amount first. Try a few drops of tincture or a spoonful of infusion taken internally, or do a patch test on the skin. If everything is fine, build up over a few days to the standard dose. If not, do not use the herb and try another one.
ALLERGIC REACTIONS	Allergic reactions to herbal medicines, even familiar ones such as chamomile, are rare and generally mild, but do sometimes occur. If you develop an allergic response to a herbal remedy, stop taking it or applying it externally. If you have been taking the remedy suspected of causing the allergic reaction for a long time, it is likely that some other factor, rather than the herb, is causing the allergy. Severe allergic reactions are a medical emergency and need immediate medical attention. See Allergy (p. 30) for advice on treating minor allergic symptoms.

Making Herbal Medicines

It is easy to forget when using manufactured herbal products that they contain botanical ingredients from plants that have been grown, sometimes for years, before being harvested and processed to make a finished medicinal product. Manufactured remedies are convenient, often highly concentrated, and come with a defined dosage, but they do not give you the independence or feel for herbal medicine that comes through handling fresh or dried herbs and making your own remedies. This section aims to give you the ability to harvest, dry, and prepare your own herbal remedies.

THE KITCHEN PHARMACY

At first sight, different herbal preparations can seem complicated and hard to make. Yet most remedies need only routine kitchen skills. The information given on the following pages should enable you to make:

+ Infusions
+ Decoctions
+ Tinctures
+ Infused oils
+ Topical applications
+ Powders and capsules
+ Smoothies

Before deciding on how to prepare a herbal remedy, look at the "best taken as" advice given in each herb profile. Most herbs can be prepared as infusions or decoctions, but some remedies – for example, horse chestnut and saw palmetto – need to be taken as tinctures or concentrated extracts. As a decoction, horse chestnut can irritate the digestive tract, while saw palmetto contains compounds that are poorly soluble in water-based preparations.

TIPS FOR HARVESTING AND DRYING HERBS

+ Make sure you know what plant you are picking and that you are picking the correct part.

+ Harvest aerial parts of plants on a dry, sunny summer's morning, once any dew has evaporated.

+ Dig roots in the autumn when a plant has died back.

+ Use a sharp knife or scissors to cut cleanly.

+ Avoid picking flowers and leaves that have blight or insect damage.

+ Drying is best done in a shaded, well-ventilated area or an airing cupboard. Whole plants can be hung up to dry, or material can be chopped and dried on brown paper (do not use newspaper).

+ Remove – and compost – discoloured or poor-quality dried material.

+ Once it is dry, chop or crumble the herbal material and store it in a clearly labelled glass jar or a brown paper bag.

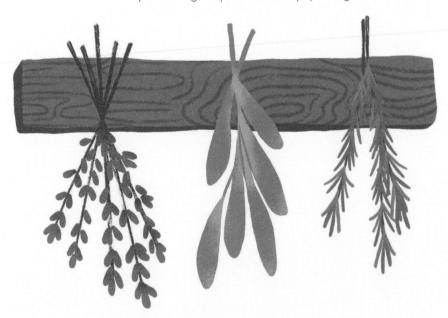

INFUSIONS

Water-based preparations, such as infusions and decoctions (see opposite), are the easiest way to make herbal remedies. Infusions are used for delicate, aerial plant parts, such as flowers and leaves. Making an infusion is more or less the same as making a tea, but herbs should always be infused in a closed container, as essential oils escape into the air if there is no lid on the pot or cup. Greater care should also be taken in terms of the quantities of plant material and boiling water used. Dried herbs are more concentrated than fresh herbs, so you will need smaller amounts. Fresh herb material tends to have a lighter, less intense effect. The quantities given here are for using dried herbs; if you are using fresh herbs, simply multiply the quantities by one and a half.

MAKING AN INFUSION

10 g (⅓ oz) dried herb
200 ml (7 fl oz) water

1. Using a glass or ceramic pot or cup with a lid, put the loose herb material in the pot and pour on water just off the boil. Stir and cover.

2. Brew for 10 minutes, then strain. To increase astringency – for example, to treat a sore throat – infuse for longer, perhaps 15 minutes.

3. Drink the infusion as two or three doses and use within 24 hours. An infusion is best kept in a refrigerator once cool.

FOR EXTERNAL USE

Besides drinking, infusions can be used as hand and foot baths. Make a 200 ml (7 fl oz) standard infusion, strain, place it in a suitable pan or bowl, and add an additional 200 ml (7 fl oz) of hot water. Soak hand(s) or feet in the bath for 10 to 15 minutes, topping up with hot water if needed.

DECOCTIONS

Decoctions are ideal for tough plant material such as bark, roots, and berries and differ only from an infusion in that the herb material is simmered for 20 minutes, as bark and roots require stronger treatment to free active compounds. The quantities given here are for using dried herbs; if you are using fresh herbs, simply multiply the quantities by one and a half.

MAKING A DECOCTION

10 g (⅓ oz) dried herb
300 ml (10½ fl oz) water

1. Using a small ceramic or stainless-steel pan, put the chopped herb material in the pan and pour freshly boiled water into the pan.

2. Simmer gently for 20 minutes, allowing the steam to escape.

3. Strain the decoction and drink it as two or more doses, using all of it within 48 hours. Keep it in a refrigerator once cool.

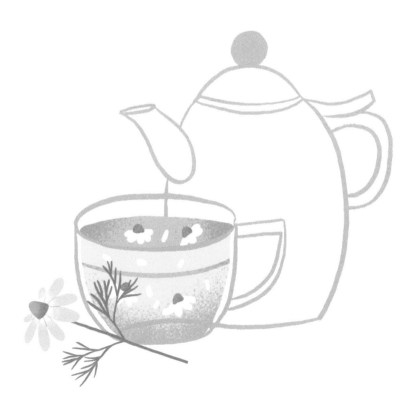

TINCTURES

Tinctures are stronger than infusions or decoctions because they extract both water-soluble and alcohol-soluble compounds within the plant. This means they have a wider therapeutic activity and are taken at a lower dosage than infusions or decoctions. Always use alcohol such as vodka – typically 40 per cent ethanol – when making a tincture. Never use other types of alcohol, such as industrial alcohol and methanol, which are highly toxic.

Extracts can also be prepared using vinegar or glycerol rather than alcohol. Usually, tinctures are made in different strengths, expressed as ratios. In this book, recommended tinctures are made using one part herb to three parts liquid (a 1:3 ratio). At home, most tinctures can be made at this 1:3 ratio, though very bulky herbs may need to be made at a 1:4 ratio, making them slightly weaker in strength.

PRIME CONSIDERATIONS

There are several things you should decide in advance:

+ What herb material should you use and at what quantity?
+ What herb to alcohol ratio should you use? A ratio of 1:3 usually allows for sufficient liquid to cover the herb material and prevent mould growth.
+ What strength of alcohol should you use? With fresh herbs, it is best to use alcohol such as vodka or rum at 37.5–40 per cent (= 70 proof). If there is too little alcohol, there is a risk of fermentation and the tincture going off.

MAKING A TINCTURE

200 g (7 oz) fresh herb
600 ml (1 pt) alcohol
   at 37.5–40 per cent
   proof (vodka or rum)

1. Wash your herb, checking for bugs, and cut it finely.

2. Place the herb material in a clean, wide-necked, screw-top glass jar and cover with the alcohol, following a ratio of one part herb to three parts alcohol. Screw the lid on tightly and shake thoroughly for a minute or two.

3. Store the tincture in a cool, dark place for 10 days, shaking or stirring the contents every one to two days.

4. After 10 days, strain the contents of the jar through a nylon-mesh drawstring bag and into a jug. Squeeze out as much liquid as possible. Using a wine press rather than a drawstring bag will yield more tincture.

5. Pour the liquid into a clean, dark glass bottle with a screw top or cork. Label clearly. Store in a cool, dark place. Compost the remaining herb material. If properly stored, tinctures will last for two to three years.

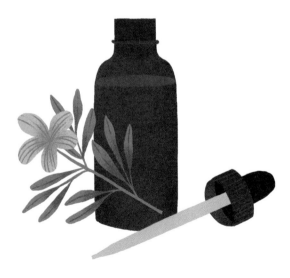

INFUSED OILS

Infused oils can be valuable when applied to the skin to promote healing and to relieve underlying pain and inflammation. They are commonly used in making ointments and as carrier oils for essential oils (see opposite). Some herbs can be cold infused. For example, fresh (or dried) marigold flowers and St John's wort flowering tops can be infused simply using sunlight. Chilli, comfrey, ginger, plantain, and rosemary can be hot-infused in grapeseed, olive, or sunflower oil using indirect heat on a stove.

MAKING A
COLD-INFUSED OIL

200 g (7 oz) fresh herb
500 ml (17½ fl oz)
  olive oil

1. Chop the herbs, place them in a clear glass, screw-top jar, and fill the jar so that all the herb is covered with olive oil. Stir and shake well, then screw on the lid.

2. Place the jar on a sunny windowsill or in a sheltered outdoor site and leave it for two to six weeks.

3. Strain the oil using a nylon-mesh drawstring bag or wine press. Pour the liquid into a clean, dark glass bottle with a screw top or cork. Label clearly. Store in a cool, dark place. Compost the remaining herb material.

4. The extracted oil can be added to fresh herb material and the process repeated to produce a stronger oil.

MAKING A
HOT-INFUSED OIL

250 g (9 oz) dried
  or 500 g (1 lb 1 oz)
  fresh herbs. If using
  hot chilli peppers use
  100 g (3½ oz) 750 ml
(1 pt 6 fl oz) good-quality
  oil

1. Chop the herbs finely, place them in a glass bowl over a saucepan of gently boiling water. Pour on the oil and stir thoroughly. Cover the bowl and simmer gently for two to three hours.

2. Allow the mixture to cool, then strain it using a nylon-mesh drawstring bag or wine press. Pour the liquid into a clean, dark glass bottle with a screw top or cork. Label clearly. Store in a cool, dark place. Compost the remaining herb material.

ADDING ESSENTIAL OILS

Adding essential oils to infused oils, lotions, creams, and ointments gives them a fragrance and increases their strength of action. You can add up to a maximum of 5 per cent of the given volume of the mixture. For example, 5 ml (1 tsp) of essential oil (approximately 100 drops) to 100 ml (3½ fl oz) infused oil, lotion, cream, or ointment. Essential oils are potent and need to be used cautiously by those with sensitive skin or who are prone to allergy. Do not add essential oils to external remedies for children under three years old.

1. Place the infused oil, lotion, cream, or ointment in a bowl with the required amount of essential oil.

2. Blend thoroughly, and pour or spoon the mixture into a screw-top glass container, and label.

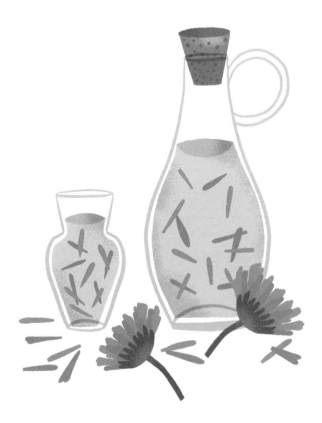

TOPICAL APPLICATIONS

Herbs can be extremely effective when used locally on the skin as lotions, compresses, ointments, and creams. A lotion is a water-based preparation, such as an infusion, decoction, or aromatic water, used to soothe or heal the skin and underlying tissue. A compress involves soaking a clean cloth in a lotion, squeezing out the excess liquid, and applying the cloth firmly to inflamed or sore tissue. Ointments are oil-based and may or may not contain water-based constituents. They tend to sit on the skin and protect and heat it. Creams are water-based and contain oils. They have a cooling and soothing action on the skin.

MAKING A LOTION

A lotion can be nothing more complicated than applying witch hazel water or aloe vera gel to the site. Different water-based preparations can be combined together as wanted, for example, equal parts of chamomile infusion and witch hazel water to soothe weeping eczema.

+ Tinctures can be diluted in water, a distilled water, or an infusion and applied as a lotion. It is usually best to use 1 part tincture(s) to 10–20 parts water (5–10 per cent tincture).

MAKING AN OINTMENT

Making an ointment is easier than making a cream. Beeswax is normally used as a natural aid to setting an ointment but you can also use oil-based ingredients, such as petroleum jelly or paraffin wax.

50 g (1¾ oz) beeswax
50 ml (1¾ fl oz) oil (olive, almond, or infused)
50 ml (1¾ fl oz) coconut oil
50 g (1¾ oz) shea butter
Optional essential oil up to 10 drops per 10 ml (2 tsp)

1. Place all the ingredients (except essential oil) in a glass bowl over a saucepan of gently boiling water.

2. As the ingredients melt, stir thoroughly until everything has liquified.

3. Slowly add in essential oils as wanted, a few drops at a time. Stir again.

4. Carefully pour into sterilized screw-top glass jars, tighten the lids, and label the jars.

MAKING A CREAM

150 g (5 oz)
  emulsifying wax
25 g (1 oz) dried herb
  or 75 g (2⅔ oz)
  fresh herb
70 g (2½ oz) glycerine
80 ml (2¾ fl oz) water
Optional small amount
  of tincture or essential
  oil up to 10 drops per
  10 ml (2 tsp)

Making a cream requires the same skill set as making mayonnaise. The art is to allow the oils you are using to blend in slowly with the water-based constituents.

1. Place the emulsifying wax in a glass bowl over a saucepan of gently boiling water (the tighter the fit the better).

2. When the wax has melted, add the remaining ingredients (excluding essential oil), stir them, and leave to simmer for three hours. Allow the mixture to cool then strain it into a separate bowl using a nylon-mesh drawstring bag or wine press.

3. Slowly add in any optional constituents and continue stirring until the cream has set.

4. Spoon the mixture into sterilized screw-top glass jars, tighten the lids, and label. Keep in a refrigerator and use within three months.

TIP Adding a 1 per cent ratio of tea tree oil will prevent mould growth (20 drops per 100 ml/3½ fl oz).

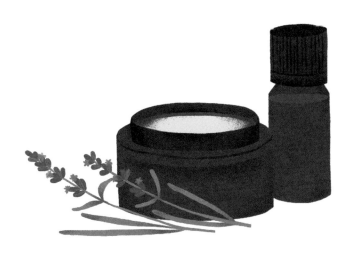

POWDERS

Powders can be blended together and are a convenient way to take many herbs, especially if placed in capsules. Dried leaves, bark, and roots can be ground at home in a coffee grinder, though industrially produced powders will be a finer grind and more consistent in size.

You can make capsules individually by hand or by using a capsule tray. Capsule shells come in several sizes, the most common being size 00, which holds about 250 mg when tightly filled. Place the bottom half of each capsule shell in the tray and fill it with powder, packing as tightly as possible. Once the bottom half of the capsule shell is full of powder, place the top half of the capsule shell – the cap – over the top of the bottom half to close the capsule. Keep your capsules in a labelled airtight container.

A powder needs to be stored in a closed container in a refrigerator – once ground, they have a very large surface area and oxidize more quickly than chopped dried herbs.

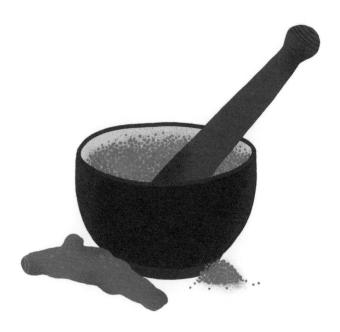

SMOOTHIES

Adding fresh or powdered herbs, or small quantities of tincture, to a smoothie is one of the easiest and most pleasant ways to take herbs.

MAKING A BREAKFAST SMOOTHIE

Choose several fresh herbs and/or powders to create your own tailored remedy. Select fruit and vegetables for taste and nutritional value, roughly chop them, and place them in a blender. Add your chosen herbs and powders and top up with water, coconut water, or milk. Blend again.

2 g (1 tsp) ginger powder
2 g (1 tsp) maca powder
2 g (1 tsp) fresh rosemary leaves
1 large carrot
1–2 sticks celery
1 apple or pear
Dash of fresh lemon juice
Water as wanted

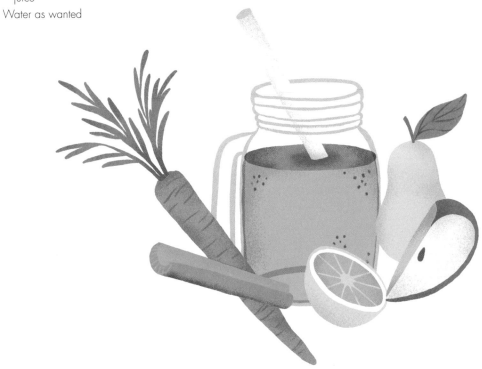

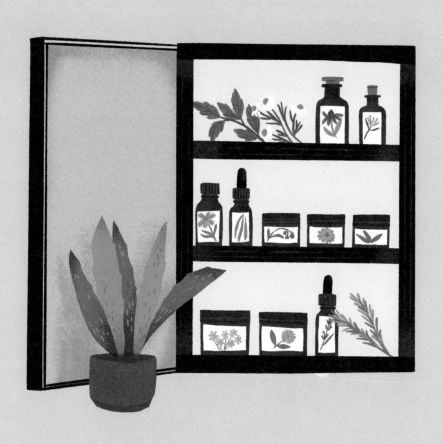

YOUR HOME HERBAL MEDICINE CHEST

Building up a herbal medicine chest, alongside a regular first-aid kit, can be a rewarding activity. Over time, you will have the resources to treat common health problems and minor injuries, as and when they happen. Aloe vera, the ultimate first-aid plant, is a good place to start. Place it on a sunny windowsill. If you have a garden or balcony, growing fresh herbs such as lemon balm, sage, and thyme will increase the range of herbal medicines available for use, as and when they may be needed. Many remedies are likely to be in your kitchen already: olive oil, lemon, honey, ginger, turmeric, pumpkin seeds, dried fruit, garlic, and onions, to name but a few.

TIP To extract your own aloe vera gel, remove a leaf from the plant and cut it open down middle. Simply scrape out the clear gel inside the leaf and apply directly or as a compress.

ESSENTIALS FOR EXTERNAL USE

+ **Marigold cream or ointment** Apply to sore and inflamed skin, acne, athlete's foot, bites and stings, minor burns, chilblains, cold sores, cuts, grazes, and minor wounds, sore nipples, and styes. It is good for children's ailments such as cradle cap and nappy rash.
+ **Arnica cream or ointment** For backache, bruises, joint pain, muscle aches, sprains.
+ **Aloe vera gel** Apply to acne, bites and stings, burns, sunburn, chilblains, cuts, grazes, and minor wounds.
+ **Comfrey, plantain, or yarrow ointment** For bruises, sprains, and fractures, to speed repair of damaged tissue.
+ **Myrrh tincture** Use neat (it will sting!) or diluted in water (equal parts) as an antiseptic to cleanse cuts, grazes, and minor wounds and prevent infection. Note: Myrrh tincture is 90 per cent alcohol.
+ **Witch hazel distilled water** Apply as a lotion or compress to inflamed and tender skin, including weeping eczema; minor burns; painful, distended veins or haemorrhoids; as an eyewash for sore eyes; and to clear "things in the eyes".

+ **Clove** Apply one drop of neat oil to the site of the toothache and on mouth ulcers.
+ **Tea tree** Apply neat oil sparingly to acne, athlete's foot, cold sores, infected bites, stings, rashes, and warts. It can be diluted in a carrier oil such as olive or coconut oil.
+ **Lavender** Apply neat oil to minor burns, bites, and stings, cold sores, cuts, and grazes, earache (one drop in the ear canal), headaches (massage sparingly into temples); apply diluted oil (5 per cent) in a carrier oil for backache, muscle aches, and period pains.
+ **Infused oils** St John's wort, grapeseed oil, or sunflower oil, as a carrier oil to dilute essential oils.

ESSENTIALS FOR INTERNAL USE

The herbs you choose to stock in your herbal medicine chest will come down to your personal choice and will depend on many factors – on your general health and well-being, on your tendencies towards ill health, whether you have children, health problems faced by family members, your age, and so on. You also need to think about how frequently you are likely to use the herbs you plan to purchase, and in what form. Tinctures, essential oils, and tablets have a much longer shelf life than dried or powdered herbs. Here are some suggestions for herbs that are always good to have at hand:

+ Chamomile: dried herb or tincture
+ Chia seed: ground when needed
+ Cranberry extract: in capsules or as a powder
+ Echinacea: tincture or tablets
+ Elderberry: extract or tincture, or dried elderflowers
+ Eucalyptus: dried herb or essential oil
+ Meadowsweet: dried herb or tincture
+ Peppermint: dried herb or essential oil
+ St John's wort: infused oil
+ Thyme: dried herb, tincture, or essential oil

THE MEDICINE GARDEN

Few pastimes are more rewarding than growing your own herbs for use as food and medicine, and there are herbs, such as marigold and rosemary, that will grow with ease in a garden, a pot on a balcony, or in a window box. Most medicinal plants require little more than a sunny aspect, adequate water, and soil and, as a rule, they prefer a little neglect to being over-tended. Whether you choose to grow from seed or cuttings, or buy established plants, in a short time you will have a quiet corner in your life that can bring flavour to your food, and health and well-being to body, mind, and soul.

There is almost no limit to the number of medicinal plants that you can grow, given a little ingenuity and determination, but the herbs listed below are some of the best to begin with:

+ Marigold
+ Chamomile
+ Echinacea
+ Californian poppy
+ Fennel
+ St John's wort
+ Lavender
+ Lemon balm

+ Nettle
+ Peppermint, mint
+ Passion flower
+ Plantain
+ Rosemary
+ Sage
+ Dandelion
+ Thyme

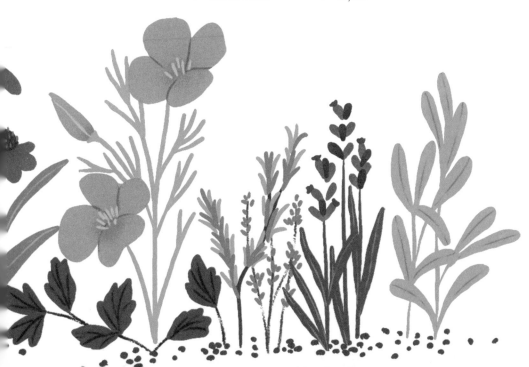

Consulting a Herbal Practitioner

As discussed throughout this book, if you think you might be seriously ill, please contact your healthcare provider whether that is a herbal practitioner, a naturopath, or a medical professional. They will be best placed to recommend treatment, should you need it. And, of course, if you have any of the "red flag" conditions listed on pp. 22–23, you must seek immediate medical attention.

Even in non-serious situations, it is always a good idea to have an experienced healthcare professional who you can contact as and when is needed. If you have a herbal practitioner, they are likely to encourage and support you in using herbs to treat yourself, family members, and friends, as well as providing professional advice and treatment. Herbal practitioners (or phytotherapists) are trained, often at university, to use their in-depth knowledge of herbal medicine to assess and treat a wide range of health problems. They are able to give detailed advice on the best remedies and products to use, together with appropriate suggestions for diet and lifestyle. A first consultation usually lasts an hour. In the UK, you can find herbal practitioners through the following organizations:

College of Practitioners of Phytotherapy
www.thecpp.co.uk

National Institute of Medical Herbalists
www.nimh.org.uk

Herbal Alliance www.herbalalliance.uk

Further Reading

Publications

Bruton-Seal J and Seal M, *Hedgerow Medicine*, Merlin Unwin Books, UK, 2008

Bruton-Seal J and Seal M, *Kitchen Medicine*, Merlin Unwin Books, UK, 2010

Chevallier A, *Encyclopedia of Herbal Medicine*, Dorling Kindersley, UK, 2023

Chevallier A, *Herbal Remedies*, Dorling Kindersley, UK, 2007

Darrell N, *Essential Oils: A concise manual*, Aeon Books, UK, 2022

Duke J, *Anti-ageing Prescriptions*, Rodale, USA, 2003

Easley T, and Horne S, *Modern Herbal Dispensatory*, North Atlantic Books, USA, 2016

Groves M, *Grow Your Own Herbal Remedies*, Storey Publishing, USA, 2019

Guyett C, *The Herbalist's Guide to Pregnancy, Childbirth and Beyond*, Aeon Books, UK, 2022

Hoffmann D, *Herbs for Healthy Aging* (USA, Healing Arts Press, 2014)

McIntyre A, *The Complete Woman's Herbal*, Holt, UK, 1995

Romm A, *Naturally Healthy Babies and Children*, Celestial Arts, USA, 2003

Stobart A, *The Medicinal Forest Garden Handbook*, Permanent Publications, UK, 2020

Useful Websites

American Botanical Council
www.herbalgram.org

Aviva Romm
www.avivaromm.com

College of Practitioners of Phytotherapy
www.thecpp.uk

Henriette's Herbal Homepage
www.henriettes-herb.com

Herb Society UK
www.herbsociety.org.uk

Herb Society USA
www.herbsociety.org

Herbal Reality
www.herbalreality.com

National Institute of Medical Herbalists
www.nimh.org.uk

Index of Herbs

Herb Profiles

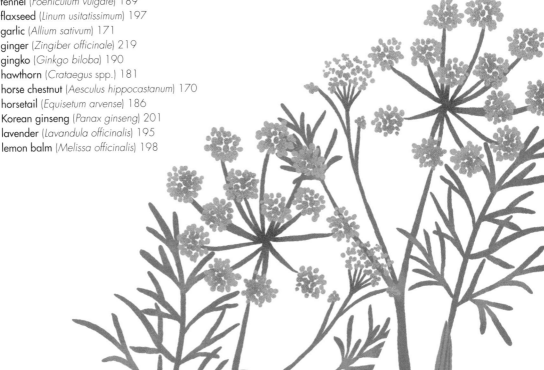

Index

Page references in **bold** indicate the main entry for the topic

Author Acknowledgements

As a herbal practitioner, one learns all the time from one's patients. Professional updates and research papers widen and deepen understanding and bring fresh insight, but over time, feedback from patients establishes a different type of understanding of herbal medicine, based on cumulative experience and the application of herbs in a practical context. In writing *The Home Herbal*, I have tried to draw especially on this area of practical knowledge and want to acknowledge the wisdom and understanding my patients have given me over the years – without them I would not have been able to write a book such as this.

My profound thanks go to Zara Anvari at DK, who had the general idea for the book, to Sophie Blackman at DK, who was key to carrying through the project to its conclusion, and to those who have been involved in the production of such a beautifully designed book: Lucy Sykes-Thompson and Barbara Zuniga. Special thanks also to Anna Southgate, who sensitively edited my text, making it seem like a smooth and simple process, and to Marisol Ortega, whose delightful, gently understated illustrations so successfully counter-balance the text.

Lastly, with warm appreciation, to friends, patients, and colleagues who took time from busy lives to read and critically comment on the final draft of the text: my thanks to Kofi Busia, Nikki Darrell, Rowan Hamilton, Gabriel Mojay, Anne Roy, Jane Thompson, and Bill Willis.

A NOTE ON GENDER IDENTITIES

DK recognises all gender identities, and acknowledges that the sex someone was assigned at birth based on their sexual organs may not align with their own gender identity. People may self-identify as any gender or no gender (including, but not limited to, that of a cis or trans woman, of a cis or trans man, or of a non-binary person).

As gender language, and its use in our society, evolves, the scientific and medical communities continue to reassess their own phrasing. Most of the studies referred to in this book use "women" to describe people whose sex was assigned as female at birth, and "men" to describe people whose sex was assigned as male at birth.

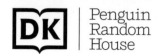

Senior Editor Sophie Blackman
Senior Designer Barbara Zuniga
Senior Acquisitions Editors Zara Anvari and Becky Alexander
Production Editor David Almond
Senior Production Controller Stephanie McConnell
Jacket and Sales Material Coordinator/Assistant Editor Jasmin Lennie
Editorial Manager Ruth O'Rourke
Art Director Maxine Pedliham
Publishing Director Katie Cowan

Editor Anna Southgate
Designer Studio Polka
Illustrator Marisol Ortega
Proofreader Francesco Piscitelli
Indexer Ruth Ellis

First published in Great Britain in 2023 by
Dorling Kindersley Limited
DK, One Embassy Gardens, 8 Viaduct Gardens,
London, SW11 7BW

The authorised representative in the EEA is
Dorling Kindersley Verlag GmbH. Arnulfstr. 124,
80636 Munich, Germany

Text copyright © Andrew Chevallier 2023
Illustration copyright © Marisol Ortega 2023
A Penguin Random House Company
10 9 8 7 6 5 4 3 2 1
001–335962–Dec/2023

A CIP catalogue record for this book is available from the British Library.
ISBN: 978-0-2416-2487-6

Printed and bound in China

www.dk.com